医学英语新医科课程群系列教材

英文医学学术论文写作

English Medical Academic Paper Writing

主　编　殷红梅　张洪芹　鲁显生
副主编　姜琳琳　卢　鹿

南京大学出版社

图书在版编目(CIP)数据

英文医学学术论文写作:英文 / 殷红梅,张洪芹,
鲁显生主编. — 南京:南京大学出版社,2021.1(2024.7重印)
ISBN 978 - 7 - 305 - 23932 - 8

Ⅰ. ①英… Ⅱ. ①殷… ②张… ③鲁… Ⅲ. ①医学 -
英语 - 论文 - 写作 - 英文 Ⅳ. ①R

中国版本图书馆 CIP 数据核字(2020)第 217680 号

出版发行　南京大学出版社
社　　址　南京市汉口路 22 号　　　　邮　编　210093
书　　名　**英文医学学术论文写作**
　　　　　YINGWEN YIXUE XUESHU LUNWEN XIEZUO
主　　编　殷红梅　张洪芹　鲁显生
责任编辑　裴维维　　　　　　　　编辑热线　025 - 83592123

照　　排　南京南琳图文制作有限公司
印　　刷　南通印刷总厂有限公司
开　　本　787 mm×1092 mm　1/16　印张 13.5　字数 398 千
版　　次　2021 年 1 月第 1 版　2024 年 7 月第 3 次印刷
ISBN 978 - 7 - 305 - 23932 - 8
定　　价　47.00 元

网址:http://www.njupco.com
官方微博:http://weibo.com/njupco
官方微信号:njupress
销售咨询热线:(025) 83594756

前　言

一、编写背景与目的

近年来,随着我国科研实力的不断提高,每年在国际期刊上发表的 SCI 论文数量和影响因子明显增加,科技影响力也逐年增强。对基础医学、临床医学和公共卫生等医学专业的科研人员和医务工作者而言,用英语撰写和发表科研论文已成常态。

本书旨在使医学专业学生习得和规范撰写英语学术论文所必需的语言表达和论证能力,为课题阶段撰写论文做好准备。本书由几所知名医学科研院校的资深教授经过四年的跟进修改完成,而且经过多轮试用,深受研究生和大学生欢迎。SCI 论文在语言表达、结构布局以及论证的逻辑性等方面都有特定的要求,因此,本书旨在引导学习者从点到面系统地了解和掌握撰写 SCI 论文的特定要求,构建和提高对语域的敏感性和分析能力,习得和掌握国际通行的写作规范,逐渐能用学术英语撰写出表达较为准确、语言运用较为得体、符合国际规范的学术论文,从而突破发表 SCI 论文的"非质量因素",提高 SCI 论文的录用率或拓展科研国际化交流平台。

二、主要内容

本书针对医学专业国际期刊论文的特征,用简单易懂的语言系统地讲解英文医学学术论文所特有的语言要素、规范的语言表达、篇章结构布局、论证的逻辑性和写作方法技能,并辅以大量的医学期刊语篇范例分析与实践练习,其语料主要选自 SCI 论文及其他相关材料;考虑到学生专业背景不同,本书采用了语言的共核理论(linguistic common core)为编程方针,引导不同医学专业背景的研究生和大学生习得医学英语写作共同的语言特性和技能。

本教材共十二章,其中每一章节由三部分构成:1) 阐释相关理论和特定功能,帮助学习者归纳英语医学学术论文写作的规律和要求;2) 通过阅读和观察相关原语料,体会和习得医学英语写作的语言特征和规范用法;3) 相关专项练习实践。

从概念内容框架上看,本教程设计为两大模块:医学学术英语的语言写作规范(Chapters One—Three)和英文医学学术论文的语篇写作规范(Chapters Four—Twelve)。前者是学术写作的基础软件,以学术语言的词法、句法和语篇等要素为基础,侧重学术英语句法的构建、论文段落写作中的演绎思维范式和语篇推进程序,激发学生对语言层面语料的敏感性,挖掘其对以往科研经验的自省能力,为英语医学论文写作奠定必要的理论与实践基础。

第二模块是硬件,即英文医学学术论文写作部分。以 SCI 论文为语料,系统讲解了规范的 SCI 医学学术论文所特定的各种语篇结构要素(包括参考文献)的功能、组织结构、语言特点、论证逻辑及其写作方法。另外,本教程以真实的国际期刊投稿过程为例,指出国际核心期刊论文的写作问题(Chapter Twelve),旨在帮助写作者进一步体会和拓展对学术英语论文发表的深度认知及能力提升。

三、主要特色

本书两大模块循序渐进又自成体系,便于教师和学习者进行梳理和巩固。教师可以根据教学计划、教学对象的状况和需求等具体情况,灵活和系统地安排授课内容,可逐章整体讲解也可分区重点讲解,以更好地体现和发挥出各章节内容的有效性和可塑性。

本书的编写以论文撰写过程为主线,还教于生、还学于生,编写中注重师生互动、生生互动以及习得反馈,每单元除设置了生动活泼的练习外,还增设了单元回顾一栏,有利于读者对重点知识的掌控,也有利于教师及时了解学生对学习的掌控。

本书并未采用传统的句—段—篇章的编写理念,而是从一开始就给学习者开启语篇模式和思维方法的训练,使学习者了解中英两种语言在语篇层面上的文化差异,并通过理论和练习使写作者摒弃其错误的"汉译英"式处理过程,建立对目标语言的正确表达方法和途径,进行规范、有效的英语写作。教师或学习者亦可辅之以汉语例文做验证对比,收效会更好。

本书语料库主要来自近几年公开发表的 SCI 期刊,如 *the New England Journal of Medicine*,*Cell*,*Science*,*Nature*,*Lancet* 等知名医学期刊。教师可以引导学生查阅适量专业论文,与本书理念和原则做验证对比,细心研读并做相应训练,相信会有较好的收获。

四、相关课程服务

作为教学的承载,为满足师生的学习与测评需求,读者可扫描二维码,获取更多相关内容,包括但不限于:教学辅助课件、实时更新的语料库等。

本书在编写过程中参考了大量国内外写作文献。在此,我们对这些文献的编者和作者表示感谢。由于编者水平有限,书中难免有不足之处,敬请读者批评指正。

殷红梅

2021 年 1 月于中国疾病预防控制中心研究生院

CONTENTS

Chapter Nine   Results Writing

Chapter Ten   Discussion and Conclusions Writing

Chapter Eleven   Contributions, Acknowledgements and References in English Medical Academic Papers

Chapter Twelve   Common Errors in English Academic Paper Writing

References

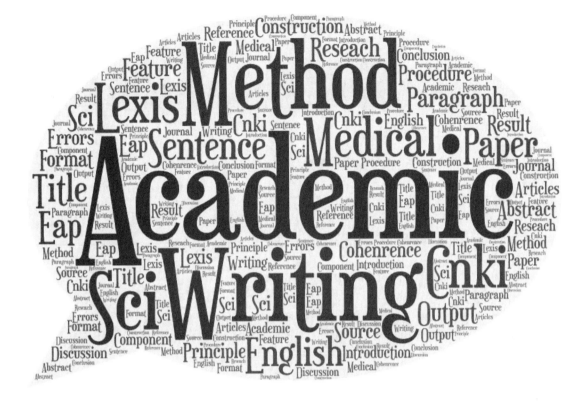

PART I

Basic Skills and Preparation for English Medical Academic Paper Writing

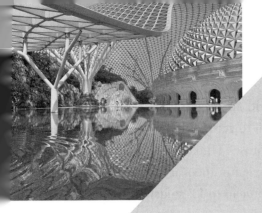

Chapter One

Lexis and Sentence Theories in Medical Academic English Writing

Lead-in Questions

1. Could you say something about the differences between spoken and academic words? Please give examples if you like.

2. Do you have any knowledge or experience about sentence types in academic English writing, especially in English medical academic paper writing?

Learning Objectives

After learning this unit, you will be able to:

1. identify the written and spoken genres of English sentences;

2. understand the lexical approach to academic English writing;

3. understand ways of constructing academic English sentences idiomatically.

✓参考答案
✓课件申请
✓学术资源

Writing is a kind of academic forms. Many second language (L2) graduates and undergraduates, after years of ESL training, often fail to recognize and appropriately use the conventions and features of academic written prose (Hinkel, 2004). Generally they employ largely conversational linguistic features even in their academic writings. So the teaching and learning of academic writing are crucial to L2 students, especially postgraduates of medical majors.

1.1 Introduction to written and spoken genres

A genre is the subject matter or category that writers use, and is generally in terms of spoken and written forms, as listed in Table 1-1. A genre is word choices and usages and vital to EFL (English as a Foreign Language) and academic writing.

Table 1-1 Written and spoken genres

Written genres		Spoken genres	
Research articles	Book reviews	Lectures	Student presentations
Conference abstracts	Ph. D. dissertations	Seminars	Office hour sessions
Grant proposals	Textbooks	Tutorial sessions	Practicum feedback
Undergraduate essays	Reprint requests	Peer feedback	Dissertation defenses
Submission letters	Editor response letters	Colloquia	Admission interviews

[Sample 1]

My dad says these are the best days of my life—but I am not so sure! You know, I've got lots of work to do and there's not much time really. I also play football for the school team and we have to do training three nights a week.

[Sample 2]

The study was conducted in three successive stages: first, we investigated the influence of climate on the temporal variation of AI incidence by measuring the correlation between AI incidence and climate variables in regions of the country characterized by different climates. Then, in order to investigate whether other factors could explain AI seasonality, we used a finite mixture mode to identify periods of time during which AIO frequency increased. Finally, we tested the influence of other factors using stochastic compartment modeling (Delabouglise et al., 2017).

[Analysis]

The two samples are different in style: Sample 1 is spoken while Sample 2 is written. First, the sentence type is different. The three sentences in Sample 1 are compound in structure（并列句）with coordinate conjunctions like "but", "and". Second, they are also different in topics（话题）：pronouns as topic in Sample 1 like "I", "my" and "we"（as topics of life activities）, content as topic in Sample 2 like "study", and "we"（as topics of scientific papers）. Therefore, Sample 1 is subjective and Sample 2 is objective.

1.2　The conventions of academic English lexis choices

Academic English writing achieves its formality through the use of specialist vocabulary, impersonal voice, and the ways that ideas get packed into relatively few words. "These features of academic writing break down into three key areas: high lexical density, high nominal style, impersonal constructions."（Hyland, 2006）It is vital and significant to master important disciplinary genres and the competence of their users in various related fields. （Hyland, 2006）Vocabulary approach is a common core, a set of language forms or skills in academic English writing.

Language consists of grammaticalised lexis—not lexicalized grammar（Lewis, 1993）. The lexical approach is a method of teaching foreign languages described by Michael Lewis in the early 1990s. The basic concept on which this approach rests is the idea that an important part of learning a language consists of being able to understand and produce lexical phrases as chunks. Students are thought to be able to perceive patterns of language（grammar）as well as have meaningful set uses of words at their disposal when they are taught in this way. In this approach vocabulary is prized over grammar. The teaching and learning of chunks and set phrases has become common in English as a foreign or second language.

1.2.1　Chunk models in EAP

Chunks（语块）other than words and sentences are seen as central to language. Chunks, a typical feature of EAP（English for Academic Purposes）, take various forms like subject, predicate, object, prepositional, adverbial chunks, etc. whose major components are nouns as in Samples 3 and 4.

[Sample 3]
After the women were enrolled, *detailed demographic*, *medical*, *and prenatal history information*, as well as *clinical findings*, were entered into case-report forms. （Subject chunks of nouns）

[Sample 4]
We recorded *age*, *sex*, *socioeconomic status*, *lifestyle factors*, *current medications*, and *medical history*. （Object chunks of nouns）

This high degree of resistance severely limits *treatment options*, *necessitating the use of complex*, *toxic*, and *costly regimens*. (Object chunks of nouns)

[Sample 5]

Mexico recently introduced its National Strategy for Overweight, Obesity and Diabetes, which includes health education, improved opportunities for exercise, taxation of sugary drinks and high-calorie foods, and earlier identification and monitoring of risk factors, including diabetes. However, despite whatever is achieved in the next few decades by lifestyle interventions (e. g. with respect to adiposity, exercise, and smoking), diabetes will still affect many people in Mexico and will require treatment to reduce the risk of premature death.

[Sample 6]

Health care delivery can target both diabetes itself and other determinants of the risk of death or disability from the many different diseases that diabetes can cause. In this middle income country with a high prevalence of over-weight and obesity and with insufficient control of blood glucose, blood pressure, and cholesterol levels, diabetes was a cause of at least one of third of all deaths between 35 and 74 years of age (twice the current indirect estimates for Mexico), with the excess mortality attributed chiefly to renal disease, vascular disease, infection and acute diabetic crises. (Alegre-Diaz et al. , 2016)

[Analysis]

There are two types of lexical chunks in Samples 5 and 6, preposition-object and verb-object.

Preposition-object chunks, like "(for) Overweight", "Obesity" and "Diabetes" (Sample 5); "(with respect to) adiposity", "exercise", and "smoking" (Sample 5); "(with insufficient control of) blood glucose", "blood pressure", "cholesterol levels" and "diabetes" (Sample 6).

Verb-object chunks like "(includes) health education", "improved opportunities (for) exercise", "taxation of sugary drinks" and "high-calorie foods" (Sample 5), and "earlier identification" and "monitoring of risk factors" (Sample 5); "attributed chiefly to renal disease, vascular disease", "infection and acute diabetic crises" (Sample 6).

1.2.2 Collocations of de-lexicalized verb models of academic English writing

Lexical patterns can be more powerfully generative as collocations than structural patterns. Collocations of de-lexicalized verbs, such as "have", "make", "do", "get", "put", and "take", are often used as pattern generators, as shown in Table 1 – 2 below with corpus data newly retrieved.

Table 1 - 2   Collocations of private verbs

Private verbs	Collocations in RAC academic corpus （英国皇家科学学会学术语料库）	Collocations in BNC medical corpus （英国国家医学语料库）
do	individual counseling, correction, studies in, business, this certificate for, some translation, research in, career in research, exchanges with worldwide schools, a doctorate in communication in UQAM, tests, my inscription, many interviews, presentations	analysis, something detrimental, necessary research, difficult surgery, rhinoplasty（鼻整形手术）, a liver transplant, right acts, good rather than bad
get	permission（to）, unemployment insurance, promoted or retired, a conclusion, the indexes	an estimate, authority from, a continuing working relationship with, access to any local university, discovery/report/advice/recommendation from, some benefit, a decisive determination, a release of, discovery from, guidance as to, a lifelong conviction
take	advantage of, control of, turns, shortcuts, vote/poll/survey, the advice	the coronavirus epidemic, measures to control malaria epidemic, responsibility for decision, the intermediate view, full instructions on, possession of, installation of machinery, the consequences of, priority, account of, foodborne diseases prevention, reasonable precautions to maintain the health and safety of the current society
put	into analysis, language into use	trust, faith, or confidence in someone or something; time, strength, or energy into an activity; in place a community medical care mutual help program; forward an approach; on respirator; a premium on health insurance

［Sample 7］

We did a secondary analysis of the most recent Demographic and Health Survey data from 28 LMICs where both tobacco use and HIV test data were made publicly available.

［Sample 8］

Few of these studies make comparison with the general population prevalence or that among HIV-negative individuals.

［Sample 9］

Future interventions should take account of these complex social, psychological, and other health challenges faced by most people living with HIV.

1.2.3 Non-adjacent construction models of academic English writing

Non-adjacent constructions can be typically demonstrated by various types like subject predicates, compound predicates, predicate objects, and verbal phrases. Among them, subject predicates are most frequently used in academic discourses.

[**Sample 10**]

These data, coupled with the relatively low seroprevalence of Ad3 as compared with Ad5 worldwide, support the advanced development of this vaccine for the prevention of EVD.

[**Sample 11**]

The bivalent vaccine reported here is composed of glycoprotein constructs from two Ebola species (Zaire and Sudan), but since the Zaire species of ebolavirus was responsible for the 2014 epidemic, a monovalent cAd3-EBO Zaire vaccine (cAd3-EBOZ) was also prepared.

[**Analysis**]

Samples 10 and 11 are from *N ENGL J MED 376：10* (Ledgerwood et al., 2017). Sample 10 contains one example of non-adjacent construction like "coupled with the relatively low seroprevalence (血清阳性率) of Ad3 as compared with Ad5 worldwide", which separates the subject "these data" from the predicate "support". In Sample 11, "reported here" separates the subject "The bivalent vaccine" from the predicate "is composed".

1.3 Introduction to sentence classification in general

1.3.1 Sentential types from construction

Generally, there are four types of sentence structure in a paragraph: simple sentences, complex sentences, compound sentences, and compound-complex sentences.

A simple sentence contains one subject + one predicate-verb, but it may contain more than one subject, verb, attribute or adverbial as in Sample 12.

[**Sample 12**]

The prevalence of asthma and allergic diseases is disproportionately distributed among different populations, with an increasing trend observed in Western countries.

A complex sentence contains one main clause and one or more dependent clauses, with a connective word denoting the relation between the two parts. As a rule, the major idea is expressed in the main clause and the idea or ideas of lesser importance in the subordinate clauses as in Sample 13.

[Sample 13]

This rising trend is attributed to regions that are becoming more urbanized and westernized.

A compound sentence consists of two or more independent clauses (or simple sentences) related to each other in meaning and linked by a coordinating conjunction (and，but，or，etc.) or by a semicolon without a conjunction as in Sample 14.

[Sample 14]

The situation is very different for species that are projected to suffer extensive range losses; these are largely caused by direct human land-use change.

A compound-complex sentence，like Sample 15，contains at least two main clauses and at least one dependent clause.

[Sample 15]

Approximately 1 million people die every year from HBV-related end-stage liver disease; the burden is concentrated in resource-poor settings，including West Africa，where more than 70% of cases of hepatocellular carcinoma in people younger than 50 years are caused by HBV.

Each paragraph in an academic paper not only needs to combine the above four sentence patterns correctly in syntax，but also needs to describe and express the research information accurately and coherently.

[Sample 16]

Beginning in December，2019，a cluster of cases of pneumonia with unknown cause was reported in Wuhan，in Hubei province of China. On Jan 7，2020，a novel coronavirus，severe acute respiratory syndrome coronavirus 2 (SARS-CoV-2; previously known as 2019-nCoV)，was identified as the causative organism by Chinese facilities via deep sequencing analysis of patients' respiratory tract samples. SARS-CoV-2 has been shown to infect human respiratory epithelial cells through an interaction between the viral S protein and the angiotensin converting enzyme 2 receptor on human cells; thus，SARS-CoV-2 possesses a strong capability to infect humans. (Shi et al.，2020)

1.3.2   Sentential types from informational content

Sentences convey information for communication. A sentence with less information is called a loose sentence(松散句)，and one with more information is a compact sentence (紧凑句).

Loose sentences usually convey one concept of information in one grammatical unit.

Compact sentences generally convey more information in a single grammatical structure especially a clause or a phrase. A common violation of conciseness is the presentation of a single complex idea, step by step, in a series of sentences which might be combined into one.

[**Sample 17**]

In this single-center, double-blind, placebo-controlled, parallel-group trial, pregnant women between 22 and 26 weeks of gestation were recruited into the Copenhagen Prospective Studies on Asthma in Childhood pregnancy cohort. Women taking more than 600 IU of vitamin D per day and women with any endocrine, heart, or kidney disorder were excluded. The trial was approved by the local ethics committee and the Danish Data Protection Agency. Both parents of each child provided spoken and written informed consent before enrollment. (Bisgaard et al., 2016).

[**Analysis**]

All sentences in this paragraph are compact sentences. The first sentence contains 8 ideas (separated by//), like "In this single-center//double-blind//placebo-controlled// parallel-group trial//pregnant women//between 22 and 26 weeks of gestation//were recruited into the Copenhagen Prospective Studies//on Asthma in Childhood pregnancy cohort"; the second one has 5 units of information like "Women taking more than 600 IU of vitamin D//per day//and women with any endocrine//heart, or kidney disorder//were excluded"; the third one has 4 units of information like "The trial//was approved//by the local ethics committee//and the Danish Data Protection Agency"; and the last one has 4 ideas like "Both parents of each child//provided spoken//and written informed consent//before enrollment."

1.3.3　Sentential types from style

Sentence types from style can be divided into two types: spoken and written sentences. Spoken sentences are commonly found in informal contexts like spoken communication. Two obvious features are found in spoken sentences: a) animate subjects (人称主语句) like "I/You/think/suppose/believe/..."; b) a loose structure with less information conveyed like "If he finishes the experiment, he will finish writing the paper in time".

Written sentences are generally used in formal contexts like written communication. Two obvious features are found in written sentences: a) inanimate subjects (非人称主语句), b) compact structure with various information.

[**Sample 18**]

Early recognition may be difficult in countries such as the United States, where most physicians have never seen a case of yellow fever and know little about the clinical manifestations. Typically, yellow fever is suspected on the basis of clinical presentation and confirmed later, since definitive diagnosis requires testing available only in specialized laboratories. The clinical illness manifests in three stages: infection, remission, and intoxication. During the infection stage, patients present after a 3-to-6-day incubation period with a nonspecific febrile illness that is difficult to distinguish from other flulike diseases. High fevers associated with bradycardia, leukopenia, and transaminase elevations may provide a clue to the diagnosis, and patients will be viremic during this period.

[Analysis]

The written passage is formal in style with two obvious features: 1) inanimate subjects (非人称主语句), like "Early recognition", "yellow fever", "The clinical illness", "High fevers", etc.; 2) compact structure with various information like compact sentences in simple construction (复杂信息内容的简单句) like the long sentences in the first, second, fourth construction; and even the third part like "The clinical illness manifests in three stages: infection, remission, and intoxication" contains complex information in this sentence.

1.4　Academic English sentence constructions

1.4.1　The conventions of sentential construction in academic English writing

There are at least three key requirements of academic writing, concerning high lexical density, high nominal style, and impersonal construction (Hyland, 2006).

1.4.1.1　High lexical density

A high proportion of content words in relation to grammar words such as prepositions, articles and pronouns make academic writing more tightly packed with information.

[Sample 19]

Large-scale diagnostic testing is a key tool in epidemiology and in containing outbreaks such as COVID-19.

[Sample 20]

You can make large-scale diagnostic testing because it is a key tool in epidemiology and in containing outbreaks such as COVID-19.

[Analysis]

Sample 19 is tightly packed with information, high lexical density (a simple sentence), high nominal style (testing, epidemiology, outbreaks), and impersonal construction (Large-scale diagnostic testing), while Sample 20 is loose in information with a complex sentence structure，and a personal subject.

1.4.1.2　High nominal style

Actions and events are presented as nouns rather than verbs to package complex phenomena as a single element of a clause. This freezes an event，such as "Nucleic acid tests（NATs）can diagnose SARS-CoV-2" and repackages it as an object："Diagnosis of SARS-CoV-2 with nucleic acid". Turning processes into objects in this way can express scientific perspectives that seek to show relationships between entities.

1.4.1.3　Impersonal constructions

Students are often advised to keep their academic prose as impersonal as possible，avoiding the use of "I" and expressions of feeling. First-person pronouns are often replaced by passives（"the solution was heated"），dummy "it" subjects（"It is possible to manage the patients with COVID-19 by means of nucleic acid tests."），and what are called "abstract rhetors"（抽象主语），where agency（施事）is attributed to things rather than people（"the data suggest"）.

[**Sample 21**]

Diabetes is increasingly common in many countries and has been found to increase the risk of death from a wide range of diseases. However，most large studies of diabetes have been conducted in high-income countries where patients have access to good medical care and can receive treatments to establish and maintain good glycemic control. In a meta-analysis of 97 prospective studies，which were conducted mainly in high-income countries，self-reported diabetes less than doubled the rates of death from any cause. In contrast，in middle-income and low-income countries，where resources to manage diabetes may be more limited and vascular-protective medications may be underused，the effects of diabetes on mortality from other diseases could be substantially larger. In many such countries，the prevalence of diabetes has increased considerably over the past few decades（Alegre-Diaz et al.，2016）.

[**Analysis**]

This sample is from *N Engl J Med 2016；375：1961 - 71*. Impersonal constructions are found especially in sentence subjects like "Diabetes（is increasingly common）//most large studies of diabetes（have been conducted）//self-reported diabetes//vascular-protective medications（may be underused）//the prevalence of diabetes（has increased considerably over the past few decades）."

1.4.2　Constructions of academic sentences for L2 postgraduates

This unit shows concrete skills and examples of how to simplify grammatical structure and add information to grammatical constructions.

1. Replace compound sentences or multiple complex sentences with simple sentences.

[**Sample 22**]

When they are heated under pressure, the constituents fuse together. (a complex sentence)

→22₁ When heated under pressure, the constituents fuse together. (a simple sentence)

→22₂ Heated under pressure, the constituents fuse together. (a simple sentence)

[**Analysis**]

A complex sentence in Sample 22 can be replaced by a simple sentence 22_1 or 22_2, making its information densely packed as in 22_2.

2. Replace grammatical expressions with lexical ones.

[**Sample 23**]

The progress of the work will depend on how modern the equipment is.

→23₁ The progress of the work will depend on the modernization of the equipment.

[**Analysis**]

The noun phrase "the modernization of the equipment" in Sample 23_1 replaces the grammatical clause "how modern the equipment is" in Sample 23.

3. Condense two simple sentences into one by using a non-predicate verb phrase.

[**Sample 24**]

SARS-CoV-2 infection can be diagnosed by nucleic acid tests (NATs). These tests are typically used after the onset of symptoms.

→24₁ SARS-CoV-2 infection can be diagnosed by nucleic acid tests (NATs) <u>typically used after the onset of symptoms</u>.

[**Analysis**]

Sample 24 is loose in information while the revised sentence 24_1 is compact.

4. Combine two short sentences by using a prepositional phrase.

[**Sample 25**]

The citizens are quarantined at home because the COVID-19 epidemic is severe.

→25₁ The citizens are quarantined at home due to the severe COVID-19 epidemic.

→25₂ The severe COVID-19 epidemic keeps the citizens quarantined at home.

[**Analysis**]

Sample 25 shows a loose complex sentence structure while the simple sentences 25_1 and 25_2 are dense in structure and information.

5. Build lexical phrases to enrich sentence content.

Generally there are many phrasal types in discourse, namely n. + n. , adj. + n. , adj. + adj. + n. , adv. + adj. , adv. + adj. + n. and adv. + adv.

n. + n. : pressure and challenges; animation and puppets; relaxation and entertainment; cough, wheeze, and dyspnea; asthma, allergy, and eczema; wheeze or asthma.

adj. + n. : daily prevalence; sheer relaxation; increased mortality; complex, toxic, and costly regimens; tested blood and urine specimens; this large, prospective, multinational study of the epidemiology of acute kidney injury.

adj. + adj. + n. : a prospective, observational study; a brief, businesslike way; chronic systemic diseases; possible fetal abnormalities.

adv. + adj. + n. : statistically significant interaction; significantly diminished burden.

adv. + adj. : extremely valuable; grossly abnormal results; currently common; rapidly blinking; previously diagnosed; reasonably reliable.

adv. + adv. : currently or previously; necessarily and sufficiently; environmentally and responsibly; quickly and locally; rapidly and effectively.

[Sample 26]

There should be an increased public health awareness of differences in mental health issues between men and women. Public health interventions including education and suicide prevention efforts focused on men, especially adolescent males and young men, are needed. Men's mental health needs more attention from clinicians, researchers, and health policymakers. Medical and legal professionals and lawmakers should be better educated about the issues related to men's mental health.

[Analysis]

This academic passage contains many lexical phrases: "an increased public health awareness of differences//mental health issues between men and women//Public health interventions//education and suicide prevention efforts focused on men//adolescent males and young men//Men's mental health//more attention//from clinicians, researchers, and health policymakers//Medical and legal professionals and lawmakers//educated about the issues//related to men's mental health" etc.

6. Use paralleled structure（排比结构）to enrich sentential information.

[Sample 27]

A new law mandates that Medicare, Medicaid, other government health care and insurance plans, and most private plans cover COVID-19 testing in the United States without copays or deductibles. COVID-19 tests can be grouped as nucleic acid, serological, antigen, and ancillary tests, all of which play distinct roles in hospital, point-of-care, or large-scale population testing.

［**Sample 28**］

The uses of serological testing included determination of previous viral exposure in the population <u>for retrospective assessment of the efficacy of control measures</u>，assessment of immune status <u>for individuals</u>，and determination of surrogates of immunity <u>for vaccine development</u>. Secondary end points included analyses of vaccine efficacy <u>against rotavirus gastroenteritis</u> of any severity，<u>against very severe rotavirus</u> gastroenteritis，<u>and against gastroenteritis</u> of any cause.

［**Sample 29**］

Data were excluded <u>if the source did not record the period prevalence of diarrhea</u> for every child in the home in the preceding 2 to 4 weeks；<u>if the source did not include</u> strata，primary sampling unit，and design weights for each participant；<u>and if the source did not include geographic information</u> that was more specific than at the national scale.

［**Analysis**］

Parallelism is parallel to putting the same or similar structure，the same tone，meaning related sentences or elements together，arranging a pair or series of similar related words，phrases，or sentences. Samples 27，28 and 29 take advantage of parallelism，using parallel structure in words，phrases and sentences respectively. Parallelism at rhetorical level makes the language elaborate，the rhythm harmonious，and tones convincing.

1.4.3 Suggestions for style choices

Providing learners with greater understanding of and access to valued genres is a crucial aspect of this demystification—not least because it is students from non-English-speaking backgrounds who are among the most disadvantaged by lack of such access（Hyland，2006）.

L2 student writers tend to neglect writing styles or they habitually write spoken dialogues in their writing. Consequently，their writings show the feature of spoken features as "We assume that …" and "There is no doubt that …". Academic writing needs to reflect the characteristics of formal written language，with exclusion of spoken sentences. There are three suggestions concerning style choices below.

1. Use topics（话题）as sentential subjects（句子主语）.

Do not take "I/You" as sentential subjects，as in "And at this time，*you* have to learn how to get well with others so that *you* will not be lonely and will play with *your* friends happily." Do use "Mental health/Extensive research …" as sentential subjects.

2. Do not use modal verbs.

Do not use modal verbs like "should/must"，"may be"，"will not"，etc. in sentential construction. Do use lexical words to show modality（情态）like "be expected"，"be possible"，"be reluctant"，"tend to"，etc.

3. Do not take use of Band 4 or 6 essay samples from the Internet.

Do not take use of Band 4 or 6 essay samples from the Internet. Make frequent references to native writings especially classical essays and academic essays and research papers so as to avoid the negative transfer of Chinese language and culture.

Chapter Review

This part introduces written and spoken genres，and the lexical approach to academic English writing. The 160 most essential academic adjectives are enforced as well. The main instruction in this part is a general classification of sentence types. General suggestions regarding to style choices are finally given in this part.

1. In academic English writing，lexis takes generally two forms：
   - chunk models in academic English writing；
   - collocations of de-lexicalized verb models of academic English writing.
2. According to different criterion，a general classification of sentence types includes：
   - sentential types from construction；
   - sentential types from information；
   - sentential types from style：sentential construction in academic English writing.

Assignments

Task 1　*Try to find the three features of high lexical density，high nominal style，and impersonal constructions in the following academic text（from Projected Impacts of Climate and Land-Use Change on the Global Diversity of Birds）.*

Projected Impacts of Climate and Land-Use Change on the Global Diversity of Birds

Accelerated climate change and the destruction of natural habitats through direct human activities are two of the greatest threats to terrestrial biodiversity. In recent decades，they have led to substantial range contractions and species extinctions. Even more dramatic environmental change is projected for this century. Substantial evidence emphasizes the importance of human land-use changes as a cause of species declines and extinctions. Recent studies have highlighted existing and future impacts of human-induced climate change on species persistence and have stressed climate change as a primary concern for the setting of conservation priorities. Most of these studies have been based on data collected in the temperate zone，where climate change is predicted to be more pronounced. To state，there have been no global forecasts of the relative and synergistic effects of future climate change and habitat loss on vertebrate distributions. Moreover, our conceptual understanding of what makes some regions and species vulnerable to one threat or the other is still limited. We integrated the exposure of species to climate and land-use change through the combined effects of these drivers on global land cover and explored the resulting reductions in range size and possible extinctions within the world's 8,750 terrestrial bird species. For this first global assessment, we used the simplifying yet transparent assumption of stationary geographic ranges, which allows us to quantify risk in terms of the projected vegetation changes across a species' current range. Although this assumption yields worst-case projections and a number of factors could modify the local details and timeline of our projections, we think the general picture that emerges is robust: a clear and striking geographic disjunction between the relative impacts of future habitat loss and climate change on global avian diversity. (Jetz et al., 2007)

Task 2   *Analyze the following text by Weissleder et al. for its phrasal types and simple sentences.*

COVID-19 Diagnostics in Context
(http://stm. sciencemag. org/20200608)

COVID-19 tests can be grouped as nucleic acid, serological, antigen, and ancillary tests, all of which play distinct roles in hospital, point-of-care, or large-scale population testing. Table 1 summarizes the existing and emerging tests, current at the time of writing (May 2020). A continuously updated version of this table is available at https://csb. mgh. harvard. edu/covid. In NATs, viral RNA is reverse-transcribed into DNA, which is then amplified through polymerase chain reaction (PCR). NATs are the most widely used tests for detection of SARS-CoV-2 (the virus that causes COVID-19) and are increasingly run on automated platforms that take several hours to complete (4). The U.S. Food and Drug Administration (FDA) and Centers for Disease Control and Prevention (CDC) have recommended distinct SARS-CoV-2-specific RNA regions for testing (viral nucleocapsid N1, N2, and human RNase *P* gene), primers, and reagents (5). This assay differs from the World Health Organization (WHO) assay, which targets the CoV-2 RNA-dependent RNA polymerase (RdRP) and envelope (E) genes (6). By May 2020, more than 100 U.S. public health laboratories had completed the CDC's verification process and started offering NATs. These assays, including those from cleared commercial vendors, have high analytic sensitivity and specificity for SARS-CoV-2 if sample acquisition, preparation, and device operation are carried out by trained personnel.

Serological tests rely on affinity ligands to assess host response proteins [host immunoglobulin G (IgG), IgM, interleukins, and other host components]. Most IgG/IgM serum tests use recombinant viral proteins or peptides harvested from *Escherichia coli* or human embryonic kidney (HEK) 293 cells as capture reagents for human IgG/IgM. These tests need to accurately distinguish past infections due to SARS-CoV-2 from those caused by other human coronaviruses. The uses of serological testing include determination of previous viral exposure in the population for retrospective assessment of the efficacy of control measures, assessment of immune statue for individuals, and determination of surrogates of immunity for vaccine development. Each of these uses places different constraints on diagnostics.

Most antigen tests probe for the nucleocapsid (N) or spike (S) proteins of SARS-CoV-2 via lateral flow or ELISA (enzyme-linked immunosorbent assay) tests. These tests can be performed using nasopharyngeal swabs and take less than an hour to complete. Ancillary tests comprise a broad category of personal devices (apps and wearable sensors) and hospital laboratory tests, including blood gas analysis, coagulation tests, and indicators of cytokine storm (7) such as interleukin-6 (IL-6), ferritin, granulocyte colony-stimulating factor (G-CSF), macrophage inflammatory protein-1α (MIP-1α), and tumor necrosis factor-α (TNF-α). These tests aid in the management of patients with COVID-19.

Task 3 *Try to find the paralleled features in the following academic text from* **Nature Ecology & Evolution** (Ngonghala et al., *2017*).

The world's rural poor rely heavily on their immediate natural environment for subsistence and suffer high rates of morbidity and mortality from infectious diseases. We present a general framework for modeling subsistence and health of the rural poor by coupling simple dynamic models of population ecology with those for economic growth. The models show that feedbacks between the biological and economic systems can lead to a state of persistent poverty. Analyses of a wide range of specific systems under alternative assumptions show the existence of three possible regimes corresponding to a globally stable development equilibrium, a globally stable poverty equilibrium and bistability. Bistability consistently emerges as a property of generalized disease-economic systems for about a fifth of the feasible parameter space. The overall proportion of parameters leading to poverty is larger than that resulting in healthy/wealthy development. All the systems are found to be most sensitive to human disease parameters. The framework highlights feedbacks, processes and parameters that are important to measure in studies of rural poverty to identify effective pathways towards sustainable development.

Task 4   *Scan the QR code and read the Introduction sections of the first two SCI papers in Appendix Ⅱ, and discuss their sentence types. Consider the questions: In which context is it appropriate to use spoken and written sentences? What are the characteristics of the sentences in your study field? Are they loose or compact? Spoken or written?*

Task 5   *Write a paragraph or an essay relevant to your major, count the sentence types you frequently use and analyze the difference between your sentences and native ones. Then please make further suggestions concerning L2 sentence writing or sentence types.*

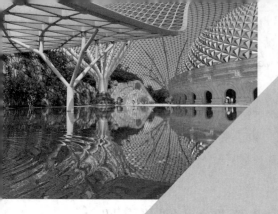

Chapter Two

Academic English Paragraph Construction Methods

Lead-in Questions

1. How are the paragraphs in an academic paper constructed?

2. What are the ways of constructing academic English paragraphs?

Learning Objectives

After learning this unit, you will be able to:

1. understand the structure of academic English paragraphs,

2. understand the logical order of constructing academic English paragraphs,

3. and write academic English paragraphs in an idiomatic way.

✓参考答案
✓课件申请
✓学术资源

2.1   Introduction to the structure and logic of academic English paragraphs

2.1.1   The structure of academic English paragraphs

A paragraph is a group of sentences that develop one central idea. An effective paragraph must be unified, coherent, specific, and adequately developed. So a paragraph is a unit of thoughts. To introduce a new thought or topic, the writer has to start with a paragraph. A standard paragraph has two important components: a topic sentence, sub-topic sentences and 5—7 supporting sentences, including 7—10 sentences in total as in Figure 2 - 1 below.

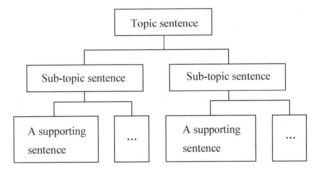

Figure 2 - 1   The logical structure of a paragraph

[Sample 1]

Our study had several limitations. First, at the time of data collection, nucleic acid testing for the diagnosis of SARS-CoV-2 infection had not yet been introduced at Union Hospital, and 33 patients were therefore diagnosed clinically on the basis of WHO criteria. However, all these cases were confirmed by nucleic acid testing when kits became available later. Second, we compared imaging patterns between four groups of different time intervals from the onset of symptoms, which does not account for potential individual variations. Third, because of the short time for case collection, follow-up CT scans were available for only 57 patients, around 40% of whom had only two CT scans. Although we have outlined the main patterns of evolution seen on CT imaging in patients with COVID-19 pneumonia, long-term radiological follow-up is needed to confirm our findings. Finally, as lung biopsy specimens were not available in this study, the relationship between radiological and histopathological findings remains to be investigated. Therefore, other potential causes of groundglass opacity, such as pulmonary oedema and haemorrhage, cannot be estimated. (Shi et al. , 2020)

［**Analysis**］

The first sentence is a topic one "Our study had several limitations". The topic sentence is supported by four sub-ideas "nucleic acid testing not yet introduced at Union Hospital", "not account for potential individual variations", "follow-up CT scans available for only 57 patients", and "the relationship between radiological and histopathological findings remains to be investigated". These subtopics are further illustrated with examples and data.

2.1.2　The logic of academic English paragraphs

Conventionally，writing needs to be arranged deductively（演绎法）as shown in Figure 2‑2. Deduction is an inference method from generalized knowledge（main idea）to case observations（supports，cases or examples）. It is a common way of reasoning in scientific study and academic paper writing. Deduction from supports to cases can be further realized by the specific methods of paragraph constructions：definition，illustration，time，space，comparison and contrast，etc. as exemplified in Sample 2.

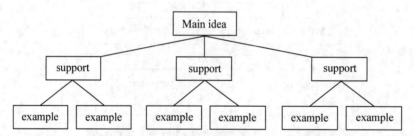

Figure 2‑2　An outline of conventional inference in academic paragraphs

［**Sample 2**］

Chronic stress is most common among people in the workplace，especially among women. Scientists studying stress in the workplace say many working women are under severe stress because of the pressures of work，marriage and children. Some experts say that pressure can cause a chemical imbalance in the brain that can lead to depression. More than thirty-million American women suffer from depression. These problems are linked to their stress-filled lives and constant hurrying. （黄一瑜、闵楠、殷红梅，2008）

［**Analysis**］

This paragraph is developed in a deductive way，with main idea conveyed by the topic sentence "Chronic stress is most common among people in the workplace，especially among women". This main idea is supported by a sub-idea，i. e. the second sentence, "many working women are under severe stress because of the pressures of work，marriage and children." And then it is further illustrated by detailed examples from experts' opinions and examples.

2.2   Academic English sentential conventions in medical paragraphs

2.2.1   The topic sentence and its function in journal article paragraphs

Generally, the topic sentence is the first sentence as in Samples 1 and 2. It may also be found in the middle or at the end of a paragraph as in Sample 3. A topic sentence summarizes the main idea of a paragraph. It tells the readers what to expect in the paragraph. Usually it is the most general and most important statement in the paragraph. The topic sentence does the following tasks: it names the topic in the paragraph, telling the readers what the paragraph is about (e. g. claimed ... lives/ strengths); it contains a controlling idea that commits the paragraph to a specific aspect of the topic (e. g. hundreds of thousands of/several).

[Sample 3]

Yellow fever most likely originated in Africa and was imported into the Americas in the 1600s. **It claimed hundreds of thousands of lives in the 18th and 19th centuries.** The Philadelphia yellow fever epidemic of 1973, for example, killed approximately 10% of the city's population and prompted the federal government to flee the city. In 1881, Cuban epidemiologist Carlos Finlay proposed that yellow fever was a mosquito borne infection. The U. S. Army physician Walter Reed and a Yellow Fever Commission verified that fact in 1900. Subsequently, mosquito-control efforts and better sanitation practices virtually eliminated yellow fever from the United States and other nonendemic areas of the America, although sporadic outbreaks of varying magnitude continued to occur in tropical regions where the disease was endemic. (Paules & Fauci, 2017)

[Analysis]

In this sample, the second sentence is the topic sentence, with the controlling ideas of thousands of casualties in the 18th and 19th centuries. All the other sentences are supporting sentences, explaining the two periods in the two centuries. And they are all relevant to the main idea.

2.2.2   The requirements of topic sentence writing in medical journal article paragraphs

There are four requirements of topic sentence writing. First, a topic sentence is affirmative (肯定句), not interrogative (疑问句) or negative (否定句). Second, a topic sentence is an opinion, not a fact. It generally contains subjective words like injurious（有害的）or beneficial（有益的）. Third，a good topic sentence has a controlling idea like "many talents", "three effects", "beneficial physically and mentally". Last，a good topic sentence is neither too broad（e. g. Diabetes is effective or common）nor too narrow（e. g. Diabetes is caused by genetic factors. ）.

【Sample 4】

Diabetes is more common and has much larger effect on mortality in Mexico than in major high-income countries. By 60 to 74 years of age，approximately one quarter of the participants in the current study had received a medical diagnosis of diabetes，as compared with approximately 7% in the United Kingdom and approximately 15% in the United States at the time of our baseline survey，and even after adjustment for other risk factors，the rate of death from any cause between 35 and 74 years of age was approximately four times as high among participants with diabetes as among those without diabetes. In contrast，meta-analyses of prospective studies from mostly high-income countries showed that person with diabetes had less than twice the rate of death from any cause as those without diabetes. (*The Emerging Risk Factors Collaboration*，2011)

【Analysis】

The paragraph begins with a topic sentence，the first sentence，and then gradually develops that statement into two main effects on mortality："four times" and "less than twice".

2.2.3 Supporting sentences and their functions in medical journal article paragraphs

In a paragraph，sentences which are used to support the main idea of the whole paragraph are defined as supporting sentences. They provide data，evidence，or supporting explanation for the main idea. All the supporting sentences should be relevant to the topic sentence，or they fail to contribute to the main idea of the paragraph，leading to digression（跑题）.

【Sample 5】

Our study has several important strengths. We have addressed the major limitations of previous studies by including more data sources and quantifying the prevalence of obesity among children. We also systematically evaluated the strength of evidence for the causal relationship between high BMI and health outcomes and included all BMI-outcome pairs for which sufficient evidence with respect to causal relationship was available. We used a beta distribution to characterize the distribution of BMI at the population level，a method that captures the proportion of the population with high BMI more accurately than other distributions. We used the best available evidence to determine the lowest-risk BMI. We quantified the burden across levels of development and estimated the contribution of demographic transition and epidemiologic transition to changes in BMI-related burden. (*The GBD* 2015 *Obesity Collaborators*, 2017)

[**Analysis**]

In this sample, the first sentence is the topic sentence in the paragraph, with the controlling ideas of important strengths. All the following sentences are supporting sentences, explaining strengths in this study. And they are all relevant to the main idea.

2.2.4　The concluding sentence and its function in medical journal article paragraphs

In western rhetoric tradition, a paragraph tends to have a natural conclusion by generalizing the main idea of the whole part. It is similar to the topic sentence in meaning but in a fresh way. Anyhow, a conclusion sentence cannot add new information to the paragraph, which will lead to failure of paragraph unity.

2.3　Principal methods of paragraph construction in academic English essays

2.3.1　Definition

Writing often involves defining words or terms so that readers know exactly what you mean by them. Definitions are useful for explaining the meaning of a word or a term that readers may be unfamiliar with or may misunderstand.

Two types of definitions are useful in academic writing: simple definitions and extended definitions. A simple definition is one that can be stated in a few words— "Fitness, for example, is a state of physical health, resulting from exercise and proper nutrition." An extended definition is longer, usually a paragraph or more, and can become the basis of a whole essay.

[**Sample 6**]

Rift Valley fever is an emerging mosquito-borne infection caused by Rift Valley fever virus (genus Phlebovirus, family Bunyaviridae), with outbreaks in Africa and more recently also in the Arabian Peninsula. However, the virus has the potential to spread to other continents. The infection is characterized by a high case-fatality rate in young animals and causes mass abortions in cattle, goats, and sheep. In human beings, Rift Valley fever presents in most cases as a mild illness with influenza-like symptoms. However, in 1%—3% of cases it progresses to a more severe haemorrhagic disease involving liver necrosis, ocular disease, internal and external haemorrhaging, and encephalitis, which could be lethal.

[**Analysis**]

A definition of an unfamiliar term typically starts with common and familiar terms. The term Rift Valley fever is first illustrated with a general explanation and then with a series of details from animals to human beings. Words or phrases often used in definition include "characterized by", "caused by", "in most cases", etc.

2.3.2　Illustration

Illustration is used to explain statements or ideas via examples, and details, specific instances. It provides examples—details, particulars, and specific instances—to explain statements that we make. Connections for illustration generally involve "in case", "illustration", "instance", "representative", "sample", "occurrence", "in occurrence of", "as representative of", "for illustration/instance", "sample for", etc.

[**Sample 7**]

GM foods are good for the environment. The damage to the environment that insecticides (杀虫剂), such as DDT, bring about is well known. The use of synthetic fertilizers on farmland leads to the eutrophication (超营养作用) of rivers and lakes all over the world. GM foods use fewer pesticides, herbicides and fertilizers, and, therefore, cause less pollution.

[**Analysis**]

Sample 7 develops the central idea of the paragraph by using examples and contrast. The first sentence states the main idea, and the supporting sentences provide contrasting details of the fertilizers' harms and of the GM foods' benefits to the environment. The explanation lies in the examples in the underlined parts concerning various fertilizers.

2.3.3　Development by time

Paragraph development in chronological order is called development by time. That is, all the events are arranged in the same order as they actually occurred. Chronological order presents ideas according to the time in which they occurred. It means that you begin with the very earliest and then progress to the most recent.

Table 2 - 1　Words & phrases often used in time sequence

sequence	progression	series	succession
evolution	advancement	subsequence	sequential
adjacent	cyclical	previously	subsequently
innovate	in sequence	in succession	in evolution
in advancement	in progression	in a subsequent way	in sequence of

[Sample 8]

The first cases of a new illness involving fever and rash that was deemed to have been caused by Zika virus (ZIKV) infection in Brazil were reported in 2014, and the presence of the virus was confirmed in April 2015. In October 2015, an unusual increase in the number of cases of microcephaly among newborn infants was reported in Brazil; this disorder was apparently linked to ZIKV infection. Here, we use routinely collected surveillance data and medical records to show how the spread of ZIKV in Brazil was associated with an increase in the incidence of GBS and microcephaly during 2015 and 2016. We also highlight the limitations of routinely collected data, which cannot yet explain, for example, why there were many fewer cases of microcephaly than expected in 2016. (Brouter et al. , 2016)

[Analysis]

The excerpt develops ZIKV infection chronologically from 2014 to 2016. Time expressions serve as major transitional signals to link all the sentences together, as "in April 2015", "In October 2015", "during 2015 and 2016", and "in 2016".

2.3.4 Development by space

Paragraph development by space is one of the commonest ways to arrange material. The physical appearance of someone or something usually calls for the organization of details into some kind of spatial relationship, (someone) from head to feet, (mountain) left to right, near to far, (building) outside to inside, etc.

Table 2 - 2   Words & phrases often used in space sequence

next to	on the opposite side	across	to the left
to the right	in front	in back	above
below	behind	nearby	beyond
in the foreground	in the background	foreground to background	
bottom to top	head to toe		

[Sample 9]

The prevalence of both risk factors declined in all regions during the period. South Asia had the largest drop in both the number and prevalence of children exposed to stunting or extreme poverty, followed by east Asia and the Pacific region. Accompanied by about a 16% increase in the population aged younger than 5 years in the region, sub-Saharan Africa had a rise in the number of children exposed to stunting and poverty, but the prevalence of the two risk factors also declined. Sub-Saharan Africa remained the region with the highest prevalence of children at risk in both years (Table 2). The findings were robust when the moderate poverty measure was used. (Lu et al. , 2016)

[**Analysis**]

This part is organized by spatial order，"from South Asia"，"east Asia"，"the Pacific region"，and "to Sub-Saharan Africa". The arrangement follows from the lowest to the highest prevalence of children at risk.

2.3.5　Cause and effect

Cause and effect essays are concerned with why things happen（causes）and what happens as a result（effects）. Cause and effect is a common method of organizing and discussing ideas.

Cause and effect paragraphs demonstrate the causal relationship between two sets of things. Trying to discover and reveal the causes or the effects of an event or action is one of the most common mental activities in our daily life. Therefore，the ability to clarify the causal relationship between two things is useful when we want to persuade or convince other people. An article may discuss both the causes and the effects of an event，but in a paragraph we analyze the causes or the effects rather than both.

Connections for cause-effect relationship are "in consequence"，"consequently"，"due to"，"thanks to"，"owing to"，"contributing to"，"in effect"，"hence"，"because of"，"result in"，"efficiently"，"effectively"，"in an effective way"，"so"，"is/are due to"，"the consequence of"，"one effect of"，"this is because"，"as"，"the effect of"，"consequent（levels）"，"therefore"，"as a result"，"for this reason"，"thus"，"as a consequence"，etc.

[**Sample 10**]

Genetically Modified Food — the Benefits and the Risks（excerpted）
（黄一瑜、闵楠、殷红梅，2008）

GM foods can fight malnutrition. In a world suffering from malnutrition，GM foods can answer the need for more nutritious food. To cite an example，Swiss researchers strove to create a rice strain that contains large amounts of beta-carotene and iron to counteract vitamin A and iron deficiencies. Malnutrition can refer to both under nutrition and wrong nutrition. People in rich and developed countries may have more than enough food to eat but still not the proper nutrition necessary to keep them healthy.

GM foods are good for the environment. The damage to the environment that insecticides，such as DDT，bring about is well known. The use of synthetic fertilizers on farmland leads to the eutrophication of rivers and lakes all over the world. GM foods use fewer pesticides，herbicides and fertilizers，and，therefore，cause less pollution.

GM foods can help medicine. GM foods can be used in producing pharmacological products through，"medical molecular farming：the production of antibodies，bio-pharmaceuticals and edible vaccines in plants." As early as 2005，Indian researchers reported the potential use of transgenic bananas in carrying vaccines against Hepatitis B. In the same year, the biotech company GTC Biotherapeutics based in Framingham, Massachusetts developed a herd of genetically modified goats that produce milk, which contains a human anti-coagulant called anti-thrombin.

GM foods are safe. The creators of GM crops are quick to assure that GM foods are safe and pose no threat to human health. GM crops are regulated by three agencies: the US Department of Agriculture (USDA), the US Environmental Protection Agency (EPA), and the US Food and Drug Administration (FDA). "The FDA ensures that foods made from these plants are safe for humans and animals to eat. The USDA makes sure the plants are safe to grow, and the EPA ensures that pesticides introduced into the plants are safe for human and animals consumption and for the environment. Meanwhile, these agencies act independently."

[Analysis]

In Sample 10, the four paragraphs demonstrate paragraph constructive methods, cause and effect, with the first sentence stating the main idea with several concrete explanations and examples.

2.3.6　Comparison and contrast

Comparison or contrast paragraphs are used to show similarities or differences between two things. A comparison paragraph focuses on similarities, while a contrast paragraph on differences. Comparison and contrast are frequently combined to give a full treatment of a topic. However, a paragraph usually concentrates only on similarities or differences, rather than both at the same time.

Table 2 - 3　Words & phrases often used in comparison and contrast

Comparison	like, similarly, in the same way, in comparison, in the likeness of, in a similar way, to bear resemblance to, similar to, in common with, both ... and
Contrast	unlike, in contrast to, on the contrary, while, nevertheless, despite, different from, although, contrary to, as opposed to, whereas

[Sample 11]

Although increased uptake of interventions and patient engagement are needed to maximize health gains, in our study, uptake of screening, linkage to care, and adherence to therapy were not big drivers of cost-effectiveness. Our baseline adherence of 80%—89%, although higher than the reported adherence of 77% to HIV treatment in sub-Saharan Africa, is lower than the reported adherence of 87%—88% to HBV treatment in North America. Our base-case estimate of 81%—83% potentially overestimates linkage to care in routine practice, because it was measured within a research study that provided reimbursement of transportation fees, clinics held in rural sites to facilitate access to treatment, active reminders about appointments, and good sensitization and counselling of screened participants. However, variations in these parameters had little effect on cost-effectiveness because low rates reduce both the impact, as well as the costs, which scale together. These losses and frailties are similar to what is seen in the HIV care cascade. (Nayagam et al., 2016)

[Analysis]

This part shows the way of development using the contrastive way via its contrastive markers like "although" and "however". Besides, comparative ways are also used by means of "than" and "similar to".

2.3.7　Deduction and induction

Deduction（演绎法）is a logical development from general to specific and induction（归纳法）is from specific to general patterns. "General to specific organization follows a direct approach. It leaves very little to the imagination of readers or listeners because the writer/speaker makes everything clear in the beginning itself. Generalizations help readers/listeners to understand the details, examples, and illustrations quickly." (Rizvi, 2005) Also known as the deductive method of organization, general-to-specific order is more commonly used than the reverse method, specific-to-general order (the inductive method).

[Sample 12]

Genetically modified foods resists disease. There are many viruses, fungi and bacteria that cause plant diseases. Plant biologists are working to create plants with genetically engineered resistance to these diseases. Unexpected frost can destroy sensitive seedling. An antifreeze gene from cold water fish has been introduced into plants such as tobacco and potato. With this antifreeze gene, these plants are able to tolerate cold temperatures that normally would kill unmodified seedlings.

[Analysis]

This sample uses the general-to-specific order to develop the paragraph by moving from a broad observation about a topic to specific details in support of that topic. First, it states the topic sentence at the beginning, continues to explain, and then goes to detailed examples for further illustration.

[Sample 13]

There is strong evidence that extreme heat leads to more aggression and violence. Newer data suggest that extreme weather events can cause stress and anxiety, exacerbating depression and other mental illnesses. Weather extremes can also adversely influence mental health. (Hunter et al., 2017)

[Analysis]

This sample uses the specific-to-general order or induction to develop the paragraph by moving from specific details about a topic to a broad observation in support of that topic. First, it goes to detailed examples for further illustration, and then states the topic sentence in the end.

Chapter Review

This chapter introduces the structure of academic English paragraphs, some chief requirements of topic sentence writing in journal article paragraphs, and academic English paragraph construction.

1. Based on structure, an academic English paragraph usually contains three sentential components:
   - the topic sentence,
   - supporting sentences,
   - and the concluding sentence.

2. There are seven principal means of paragraph construction:
   - definition,
   - illustration,
   - development by time,
   - development by space,
   - cause and effect,
   - comparison and contrast,
   - and deduction and induction.

Assignments

Task 1 *Identify the different methods of paragraph structural development and paragraph construction in the following excerpt "Stress: Personality and Gender Difference" by Cynthia Kirk.*

Stress is a condition of mental or emotional tension. Today, we tell about the effects of stress on people's health. Many people suffered mental and emotional problems after the September Eleventh terrorist attacks in the United States last year. Terrorism creates fear and fear often leads to severe stress. Studies suggest that stress can reduce the body's ability to fight disease and can lead to serious health problems. Stress affects everybody every day. It is your body's reaction to physical，chemical，emotional or environmental influences. Some stress is unavoidable and may even be good for us. Stress can keep our bodies and minds strong. It gives us the push we need to react to an urgent situation. Some people say it makes them more productive at work and gives them more energy.

Too much stress，however，can be harmful. It may make an existing health problem worse. Or it can lead to illness if a person is at risk for the condition. For example，your body reacts to stressful situations by raising your blood pressure and making your heart work harder. This is especially dangerous if you already have heart or artery disease or high blood pressure. Stress is more likely to be harmful if you feel helpless to deal with the problem or situation that causes the stress.

Anything you see as a problem can cause stress. It can be caused by everyday situations or by major problems. Stress results when something causes your body to act if it were under attack. Sources of stress can be physical，such as injury or illness. Or they can be mental，such as problems with your family，job，health or finances. Many visits to doctors are for conditions related to stress. Stress can lead to many other health problems if people try to ease it by smoking，drinking alcohol，taking drugs，or by eating more or less than normal.（黄一瑜、闵楠、殷红梅，2008）

Task 2　*Consult paragraph samples in this unit and write a paragraph related to your major with a topic sentence at the beginning，keeping the paragraph unified and coherent.*

Task 3　*Consult paragraph samples in this unit and write a paragraph with a deductive logical order and with explanations，examples，statistics as well.*

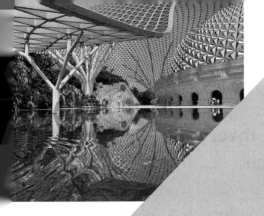

Chapter Three

Coherence in English Medical Academic Paper Writing

Lead-in Questions

What do you know about the smooth and natural running of academic English writing?

Learning Objectives

After learning this unit, you will be able to:

1. understand the theory of paragraph unity, coherence and cohesion in English medical academic paper writing,

2. master ways of constructing unified, coherent and cohesive academic English paragraphs and essays,

3. and write a logical, cohesive paragraph or essay with a unified theme.

√参考答案
√课件申请
√学术资源

3.1 Introduction to the theory of discourse coherence

Coherence is semantically meaningful in text linguistics. It is usually gained through the use of syntactical features: deictic, anaphoric and cataphoric elements, a logical tense structure, and presuppositions connected to general world knowledge as well. It is defined as the continuity of text meanings, and as the mutual access and relevance, within a concept framework of Beaugrande and Dressler (1981). Moreover, coherence is a vital term in L2 writings because of its focus upon the content and upon formal illustrations.

[**Sample 1**]

Early recognition may be difficult in countries such as the United States, where most physicians have never seen a case of yellow fever and know little about the clinical manifestations. Typically, yellow fever is suspected on the basis of clinical presentation and confirmed later, since definitive diagnosis requires testing available only in specialized laboratories. The clinical illness manifests in three stages: infection, remission, and intoxication.

During the infection stage, patients present after a 3-to-6-day incubation period with a nonspecific febrile illness that is difficult to distinguish from other flulike diseases. High fevers associated with bradycardia, leucopenia, and transaminate elevations may provide a clue to the diagnosis, and patients will be viremic during this period.

This initial stage is followed by a period of remission, when clinical improvement occurs and most patients fully recover. However, 15% to 20% of patients have progression to the intoxication stage, in which symptoms recur after 24 to 48 hours. This stage is characterized by high fevers, hemorrhagic manifestations, severe hepatic dysfunction and jaundice (hence the name "yellow fever"), renal failure, cardiovascular abnormalities, central nervous system dysfunction, and shock. Antibodies may be detected during this stage; however, viremia is usually resolved. Case-fatality rates range from 20% to 60% in patients in whom severe disease develops, and treatment is supportive, since no antiviral therapies are currently available.

Yellow fever is the most severe arbovirus ever to circulate in the Americas, and although vaccination campaigns and vector-control efforts have eliminated it from many areas, sylvatic transmission cycles continue to occur in endemic tropical regions. As with all potentially reemerging infectious diseases, public health awareness and preparedness are essential to prevent a resurgence of this historical threat. (Paules & Fauci, 2017)

［Analysis］

This is a unified essay with the central idea in the first paragraph——three stages of yellow fever, with a topic sentence at the beginning of the two supporting paragraphs as underlined. The last paragraph restates the severe effects of yellow fever in a new way. The flow of ideas occurs in a straight line from the opening sentence to the last sentence. Moreover, in each supporting paragraph there are sufficient evidence, data or supports to fully explain the central theme.

Deictic parts are: person such as "most physicians"; time such as "this initial stage", "the infection stage", "this period", "this historical threat"; place such as "the United States";

Anaphoric parts are: 15% to 20% of patients, it;

Presupposition parts are: the basis of clinical presentation, Yellow fever is the most severe arbovirus, other flulike diseases, continue to occur, this initial stage, etc.

［Sample 2］

The online competition between pro- and anti-vaccination views（excerpted）

Seven unexpected features of this cluster network（Fig. 1）and its evolution（Fig. 2）together explain why negative views have become so robust and resilient, despite a considerable number of news stories that supported vaccination and were against anti-vaccination views during the measles outbreak of 2019 and recent efforts against anti-vaccination views from pro-vaccination clusters and Facebook.

First, although anti-vaccination clusters are smaller numerically（that is, have a minority total size, Fig. 1d）and have ideologically fringe opinions, anti-vaccination clusters have become central in terms of the positioning within the network（Fig. 1a）. Specifically, whereas pro-vaccination clusters are confined to the smallest two of the three network patches（Fig. 2a）, anti-vaccination clusters dominate the main network patch in which they are heavily entangled with a very large presence of undecided clusters（more than 50 million undecided individuals）. This means that the pro-vaccination clusters in the smaller network patches may remain ignorant of the main conflict and have the wrong impression that they are winning.

Second, instead of the undecided population being passively persuaded by the anti- or pro-vaccination populations, undecided individuals are highly active: the undecided clusters have the highest growth of new out-links（Fig. 1a）, followed by anti-vaccination clusters. Moreover, it is the undecided clusters who are entangled with the anti-vaccination clusters in the main network patch that tend to show this high out-link growth. These findings challenge our current thinking that undecided individuals are a passive background population in the battle for "hearts and minds". （Johnson et al., 2020）

[**Analysis**]

This excerpt is coherent, with a deductive order such as "anti-vaccination" and "pro-vaccination", and with cohesive ties such as grammatical ties "first", "second", "instead of the undecided population" and lexical ties "vaccination", "anti-vaccination", "pro-vaccination", and "views".

3.2 Coherent conventions and thematic progression in medical essays

A paragraph has a topic sentence, supporting sentences and a concluding sentence. These sentences should lead to one central theme, with the topic sentence stating the main idea, supporting sentences pinpointing the main idea with evidence, and a concluding sentence restating the main idea in a new way. So a paragraph has the feature of unity in meaning, as in Sample 1.

3.2.1 Paragraph unity in medical journal essays

A written discourse is made up of two or more paragraphs, with a central idea called thesis statement. A well written essay is unified as shown in this chart as in Sample 1.

- Paragraph 1   Main Idea
-                  A. Sub-idea
-                  B. Sub-idea
-                  (C. Sub-idea)
- Para. 2   Sub-idea A
- Para. 3   Sub-idea B
-   (Para. 4   Sub-idea C)
- Para. 4/5   Concluding: restate the main idea

[**Sample 3**]

Understanding Depression (excerpted)
(黄一瑜、闵楠、殷红梅,2008)

Depression often looks different in men and women. An awareness of these differences helps ensure that the problem is recognized and treated.

Depression is a loaded word in our culture. Many associate it, however wrongly, with a sign of weakness and excessive emotion. This is especially true with men. Depressed men are less likely than women to acknowledge feelings of self-loathing and hopelessness. Indeed, they tend to complain about fatigue, irritability, sleep problems, and loss of interest in work and hobbies. Other signs and symptoms of depression in men include anger, aggression, violence, reckless behavior, and substance abuse. Even though depression rates for women are twice as high as those in men, men are a higher suicide risk, especially older men.

Rates of depression in women are twice as high as they are in men. This is due in part to hormonal factors, particularly when it comes to premenstrual syndrome (PMS), premenstrual dysphoric disorder (PMDD), postpartum depression, and perimenopausal depression. As for signs and symptoms, women are more likely than men to experience pronounced feelings of guilt, sleep excessively, overeat, and gain weight. Women are also more likely to suffer from seasonal affective disorder.

[**Analysis**]

Sample 3 is a unified essay because it maintains its unity by keeping the main idea of this essay in consistence with "different depression in men and women". The last two paragraphs follow the same topic "depression" and show in details how men and women are different in depression sufferings. The first paragraph states the thesis of the essay, the second explains in detail the depressions of men, and compared with men, the third paragraph explains the depressions of women. This organization can keep discourse unified.

3.2.2   Coherent conventions and thematic progression coherence in medical journal essays

Generally speaking, coherence means that the part of the paragraph is logically connected. Coherence of a paragraph is concerned with its form or its organization. The sentences in a paragraph should be arranged in a clear, logical order, and the transition should be smooth and natural. A coherent paragraph shows the features of both logical order and appropriate transitions which tie the sentences and ideas closely and smoothly via thematic progression, given and new information, and cohesion.

More specifically, the means of realizing the textual cohesion consist of grammatical cohesion, lexical cohesion and thematic cohesion. Thematic cohesion interacting with grammatical and lexical cohesion enhances the cohesion of the text and its internal information organization. The thematic organization of the text is closely connected with discourse coherence or text connection.

3.3   **Theme and rheme**

Every sentence has its own theme and rheme. From a functional point of view, theme and rheme were first proposed by Vitem Mathesius (1973), the founder and life-long chairman of the Prague School. Then, the theory of theme and rheme was developed by Halliday and other linguists (2000). "The theme is the element which serves as the point of departure of the message; it is that with which the clause is concerned. The remainder of the message, the part in which the theme is developed, is called in Prague School terminology the rheme" in Halliday's book *An Introduction to Functional Grammar*. For example,

[**Sample 4**]

A safe and effective SARS-CoV-2 vaccine may be required to end the global COVID-19 pandemic.

[**Sample 5**]

To end the global COVID-19 pandemic, a safe and effective SARS-CoV-2 vaccine may be required.

[**Analysis**]

"A safe and effective SARS-CoV-2 vaccine" is the grammatical subject in both sentences, but theme in Sample 4 and rheme in Sample 5.

Generally speaking, theme can be understood as where the speaker begins to express information and it tells people that, from this concerning point, the sentence starts its message progression. The rest of the sentence is rheme, which expresses the information that is developed from theme.

Every sentence contains a theme part and a rheme part which are definite and unchangeable in a single sentence. However, in a context or discourse, as Halliday points out, it does not mean theme definitely falls on the position at the beginning of the sentence. The position is just an assistance to realize the function of theme.

3.4　Thematic progression

Most of the discourses are composed of more than two sentences, and these sentences have grammatical or semantic relation. Moreover, they are also internally related to each other in terms of themes and rhemes. Thus the theme and rheme in the following sentences will have some connection with the theme and rheme in the former sentences.

The study of thematic progression is made mainly by Danes and Fries. Thematic progression might be viewed as the skeleton of the plot (Danes, 1974). It reflects the way of thinking of human beings. Danes finds that the connection between sentences is realized with the progression process from theme to rheme, and he thinks that it is the theme that plays an important constructing role in a context. That is to say that the real thematic progression of a discourse actually refers to the cohesion and connection of the themes, the relationships between themes and their subordinates and the relationship between themes, the paragraph, the whole discourse and the setting. All these kinds of relationships are called "the pattern of thematic progression" by Danes.

Frantisek Danes (1974) is the first person who claimed the concept of thematic progression. He postulates three main types of thematic progression: simple linear thematic progression, thematic progression with a constant/continuous theme and thematic progression with derived theme/split theme pattern.

3.4.1   Simple linear thematic progression

In this pattern, the rheme or a part of the rheme in the preceding clause/sentence becomes the theme of the subsequent clause/sentence. Danes (1974) refers to this as the most elementary or basic thematic progression. This model could be manifested in the following graph (T = theme, R = rheme):

$$T1\text{-------}R1$$
$$\downarrow$$
$$T2(=R1)\text{-------}R2$$
$$\downarrow$$
$$T3(=R2)\text{-------}R3$$

[**Sample 6**]

It (T1) all began more than three decades ago when Lovelock devised the electron— capture detector (R1). Still widely used, this electronic nose (T2 = R1) is able to sniff out a few parts per trillion of chemicals found in the soil, water or air (R2).

[**Analysis**]

In this text, the theme of the first sentence is "It"; the rheme of the first sentence is "the electron capture detector" and it becomes theme of the second sentence "this electronic nose".

In linear thematic progression, each theme naturally grows out of each previous rheme, and the paragraph coherence is achieved as themes are clearly related. With the development of theme, new content is presented to the readers one after another, so it is easier for the readers to get the main flow of the writer's ideas. In terms of writing skill, this thematic pattern can make it easier for the writer to describe or explain the object to the readers, or to emphasize the theme or rheme in a naturally logical way.

3.4.2   Thematic progression with a constant/continuous theme

In this pattern, all the clauses/sentences in the preceding and the subsequent clauses/sentences share the same theme while the rheme for each sentence is different. It could be manifested in the following graph：

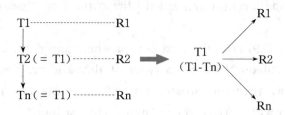

Here，rhemes describe the different aspects of the same event or thing from different angles. Peter H. Fries called this type of thematic progression theme iteration. The result of this type of thematic progression is that the themes in the text constitute a chain of co-referential items，which extend through as a sequence of sentences.

［Sample 7］

... the Gaia Hypothesis（T1）is a revolutionary idea（R1）. It（T2 = T1）argues that living things are not passive victims of their environment but can alter it（R2）. The theory（T3 = T2 = T1）could transform scientific thinking much as did Sir Isaac Newton's image of the universe as a clockwork mechanism（R3）. Gaia（T4 = T3 = T2 = T1）challenges the scientific establishment—whose experts jealously rule narrow specialties—to see a bigger picture：the world as one system in which sea and sky and life transform one another（R4）.

［Analysis］

This text is also from *The Man Who Discovered Mother Nature* by Lowell Ponte，and it provides an illustration of constant thematic progression（TP）pattern in use；here the theme of each sentence refers to the main topic of the text，the theory of Gaia Hypothesis.

3.4.3　The derived thematic progression

3.4.3.1　The derived/split themes pattern

This pattern means the meta-theme is either given in a preceding statement，or must be inferred from the common element of the sub-themes that are discussed.

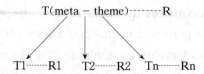

In this pattern，the first sentence is usually the topic sentence，so the theme of the first clause/sentence is often called hyper-theme of the text. The themes of other sentences are all derived from the so-called hyper-theme. In this way，theme and rheme expand separately at the same time.

[**Sample 8**]

Country-level percentage (T = T1 + T2 + T3 + T4) change in the prevalence of children at risk between 2004 and 2010 when extreme poverty measures were used is shown in figure 3 (R). Of the 141 countries assessed (T1), 123 had reductions in prevalence (R1). Among 27 countries with reduction of 20% or more (T2), 23 were middle-income countries including Vietnam (45%, the largest rate of decline), China (40%, the second largest rate of decline), and India at margin (by 20%) (R2). Six sub-Saharan countries (T3) also declined by more than 20% (Angola, Botswana, Cape Verde, Congo Brazzaville, Mauritania, and South Africa) (R3). Of the 17 countries with no change or an increase in prevalence of children at risk of poor development (T4), 11 were in sub-Saharan Africa (R4). (Lu et al., 2016)

[**Analysis**]

In this sample, the first sentence is the topic sentence, and the theme of the first sentence ("Country-level percentage") is the hyper-theme of the text. Each of the subordinate themes (T1, T2, T3 and T4) is derived from this hyper-theme and expands separately at the same time with the development of corresponding rheme. This kind of thematic progression pattern is normally used as the beginning paragraph, particularly in an argumentative, informative and explanatory text.

3.4.3.2 The derived/split rhemes pattern

This pattern occurs when the rheme of a clause has two or more components, each of which provides the theme for one or more following statements. It means that the themes in the subsequent clauses may derive from the rheme of the first clause/sentence. Like the derived themes pattern, the first sentence is also usually the topic sentence, and the rheme of the first clause/sentence is often called hyper-rheme of the text.

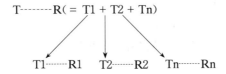

[**Sample 9**]

There are two sides to the brain(T), the left and the right (R = T1 + T2). According to one theory, the right side (T1) deals with the senses (what we see, hear, feel and smell) (R1). The left side (T2) is concerned with logic (R2).

[**Analysis**]

Here, the first sentence has a super-rheme "the left and the right". In the following sentences, each applies one side of the brain as its theme, which is derived from the original rheme of the first sentence. This kind of thematic progression pattern is frequently used to illustrate a certain point in compositions.

[Sample 10]

This study(T) has **several important limitations** (R = T1 + T2 + T3). First, the vaccine (T1) was not consistently given concomitantly with the spoken polio vaccine (R1). ... Second, the Vesikari score (T2) was originally designed for use in settings of high parental literacy, which may have led to underscoring of some cases in our trial because of low parental literacy(R2), although .... **Finally**, at the time of the analysis, no extensive genotyping data (T3) were available to weigh the vaccine efficacy against a changing pattern of circulating serotypes (R3), and ... (Isanaka et al., 2017)

[Analysis]

The super-rheme is "several important limitations" in the first sentence, which is also the topic sentence. Each of the derived themes of the following supporting sentences is taken from the super-rheme in the first sentence, explaining different aspects of the "limitations" (the vaccine, the Vesikari score and extensive genotyping data) in this study.

Chapter Review

This unit introduces the theory of coherence in academic English of medical journal essays chiefly by two sides:

1. paragraph unity in academic English of medical journal essays,
2. and paragraph coherence in academic English of medical journal essays.

Then cohesive ways are also illustrated in academic English of medical journal essays, namely:

1. grammatical transitions,
2. and lexical transitions.

Assignments

Task 1　*Read the following two paragraphs and find the irrelevant sentences in them.*

A. Only children lack companionship. An only child can have trouble making friends, since he or she isn't used to being around other children. Often, the only child comes home to an empty house; both parents are working, and there are no brothers or sisters to play with or to talk to about the day. At dinner, the single child can't tell jokes, giggle, or throw food while the adults discuss boring adult subjects. An only child always has his or her own room but never has anyone to whisper to half the night when sleep doesn't come. Some only children thrive on this isolation and channel their energies into creative activities.

B. These days the weather is getting chilly. Dressed in heavy clothes, students go back to dormitory after a day's studying. It should be an relaxing time when falling in asleep but something nettlesome change it into a nightmare. The mosquitoes are the perpetrators. Why there still are mosquitoes in such cold days? Students suffering from annoying buzz complain and wonder. In many people's notion, mosquitoes and bears alike sleep during winter. Actually, the mosquitoes are the reverse as they are still alive above 2 centigrade which means if any place indoor is warm their eggs will hatch and then become mosquitoes. So you will be annoyed by mosquitoes even in these cold days.

Task 2   *Discuss the following paragraphs in light of unity, coherence, and cohesion.*

A. In addition to being relaxing, television is entertaining. Along with the standard comedies, dramas, and game shows that provide enjoyment to viewers, television offers a variety of movies and sports events. Moreover, in many areas, viewers can pay a monthly fee and receive special cable programming. With this service, viewers can watch first-run movies, rock and classical music concerts, and specialized sports events, like international soccer and Grand Prix racing（大奖赛）. Viewers can also buy or rent movies to show on their television sets through DVD players or VCRs. Still another growing area of TV entertainment is video games. Cartridges（暗盒）are available for everything from electronic baseball to Mortal Kombat（格斗之王）, allowing the owner to have a video game arcade（视频游戏拱廊）in the living room (Langan, 2010).

B. Across mammals more broadly, the relationship between adult brain mass and longevity is accounted for by patterns of maternal investment and is generally interpreted as a manifestation of developmental costs of producing larger brained offspring, rather than necessarily due to any cognitive or behavioral mechanism. Here, however, we found that the associations of longevity with absolute and relative brain volume remain when controlling for maternal investment. Therefore, in primates, compared with mammals in general, variation in adult brain size across species cannot be fully accounted for by patterns of maternal investment, and the relationship between brain and lifespan is potentially indicative of a cognitive buffering, rather than solely developmental, mechanism through which cultural intelligence facilitates survival. This contrast can perhaps be explained by divergent scaling relationships between brain volume and neuron number in primates compared with other mammalian lineages. Unlike nonprimate mammalian lineages, such as rodents, in which neuron size increases and neuron density decreases with increased brain volume, in primates, the number of neurons increases approximately isometrically with brain volume. Therefore, in primates, larger brains may confer stronger benefits in terms of increased cognitive function and behavioral flexibility compared with other mammalian lineages. Overall, together with the strong relationship between social learning and longevity, these findings are consistent with the hypotheses that cultural knowledge facilities survival and that extended longevity facilitates the acquisition exploitation and social transmission of life skills (Street et al.).

Task 3 *Analyze the following essay in light of unity, coherence, and cohesion.*

Cognitive Changes Associated with Aging（excerpted）
（黄一瑜、闵楠、殷红梅，2008）

Research on the human brain has documented dramatic decreases in brain size and efficiency throughout our lives, beginning virtually from the time of birth. Yet, in spite of these anatomical and physiological declines, studies have found evidence of only limited decrements in actual intellectual functioning associated with the aging process. This section examines some of these known decrements in two fundamental domains of cognitive functioning: intelligence, and learning and memory.

The fact that quite a lot of older persons experience virtually no functional impairment despite their cognitive limitations is a testimony to the redundancy built into the human brain, as well as the ability of humans to find ways to compensate for potential cognitive limitations. It also reflects the fact that intellectual ability is only one of many factors affecting functioning in later life. Ultimately, intellect may be considerably less important than self-care ability and social competence in determining an older person's ability to function independently and competently, and to live a rich, rewarding life.

Intelligence

Intelligence generally can be thought of as including a range of abilities that allow us to make sense of our experiences: the ability to comprehend new information, the ability to think abstractly, the ability to make rational decisions, spatial ability, numerical ability, verbal fluency, etc. Some abilities (e. g. the ability to think abstractly) are heavily biologically determined and are relatively independent of particular applications, reflecting what has been called "fluid intelligence." Other intellectual abilities (e. g. verbal fluency) are more apt to reflect the knowledge and skills a person has gained through life experience, or "crystallized intelligence."

Intelligence tests have demonstrated a pattern of age-related changes in intellectual functioning typically beginning after the age of 60. This"classic aging pattern" involves somewhat poorer performance on tests of fluid intelligence, but little or no difference on tests of crystallized intelligence. It should be noted, however, that there is a great deal of variability in the test scores of older adults, with some older persons actually doing better than some younger persons. Moreover, older adults' intellectual functioning can be improved significantly with training and practice, although improvements generally are less than those experienced by younger persons with the same amount of training.

The factor that older persons seem to perform more poorly on tests of fluid intelligence is due in part to reduced efficiency or nerve transmission in the brain, resulting in slower information processing and greater loss of information during transmission. However, performance decrements may also be due to a variety of non-cognitive factors, including impairments in motor ability and sensation. Slower motor performance can significantly reduce an older person's ability to respond on tests that require fine hand movements (e. g. filling in the proper rectangle on an answer sheet). Sensory deficits associated with aging, for example, can result in perceptual inaccuracies, requiring the aging mind to commit more attention and cognitive effort to comprehending sensory input and reducing its capacity to quickly process new information.

Learning and memory

Most persons experience a modest increase in memory problems as they get older, particularly with regard to the ability to remember relatively recent experiences. Decrements are found both in the ability to accumulate new information and in the ability to retrieve existing information from memory storage, although there is little decline in the ability to store new information once it is learned.

The process of learning new information and encoding it for storage requires more time as individuals get older, because of the reduced efficiency of neural transmission and because of sensory deficits that limit one's ability to quickly and accurately perceive information to be learned (as discussed above). In fast-moving day-to-day experiences, this may prevent individual experiences (e. g. the name of someone to whom one is introduced) from receiving the attention needed for complete encoding into secondary memory. In addition, the extensive life experience of older persons makes it likely that new information will not adequately be distinguishable from previous learning (e. g. the names of other similar people one has met over the years), making it difficult to establish unique cues and linkages for new experiences.

Older persons also experience decrements in their ability to retrieve information once it is stored. In part, this is because of the difficulty identifying just the right piece of information from the vast store of information they have accumulated over a lifetime of experiences. This can be particularly difficult when the new information resembles previously learned information (e. g. when one is trying to recall a phone number from a thousand of phone numbers that have been learned over a lifetime). Consequently, older persons tend to do considerably worse than younger persons on tests of free recall, where they are asked to retrieve learned information but given only minimal cues. However, few decrements are found when older adults are given sufficient orienting parameters to limit the scope of the research, or are asked to select the correct answer from among a small of opinions (e. g. on a multiple choice test).

Task 4 *Write a unified, logical, cohensive essay with the topics like schoolers' depression, obesity, human disaster, healthcare, blood donation, environment risks or else.*

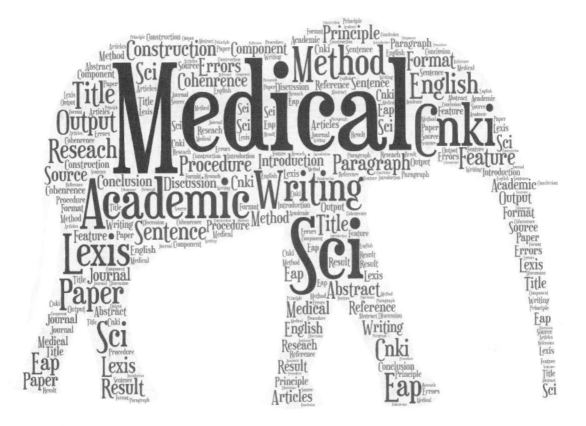

English Medical Academic Paper Writing

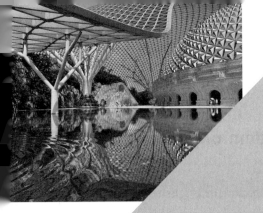

Chapter Four

English Academic Paper Writing

Lead-in Questions

1. Have you read some academic papers in English?

2. Do you have any plans to do a project and write a paper?

3. What kind of sources would you use to review the literature?

Learning Objectives

After learning this chapter, you will be able to:

1. get an overall idea about the basic procedure of medical research and English academic paper writing,

2. understand SCI and SCI papers,

3. and understand ways of topic selection.

✓参考答案
✓课件申请
✓学术资源

4.1 An overview on English academic paper writing

For scholars all over the world, writing academic papers in English and publishing them in international academic journals has become an important choice in order to make their scientific achievements more widely known and accepted. In recent years, with the continuous improvement of China's scientific research strength and capability, the number and impact factors of SCI papers published in international journals increase significantly every year, and the influence of science and technology also increases year by year. Publication in international academic journals including SCI journals has become an important symbol to measure the academic level of individuals and institutions. It has become the norm for teachers and students in medical schools, researchers in medical research institutions and medical workers in hospitals to write and publish scientific papers in English.

However, international academic journals always have their specific requirements on paper writing, especially in the following three aspects: the structural layout, logic of argumentation and language expression. Although most of the paper authors in China have more than a decade or more of English learning experience, their ability to write and express in standard academic English is still poor. Despite the good viewpoints and data of the paper, it is a pity that the paper cannot be accepted and published due to the inadequate or even incorrect expression of English language. Actually, writing and publishing academic paper in English is a challenge to most Chinese learners.

In most cases, an academic paper is both argumentative and expositive in order to share its information on a given research subject. The previous chapters have prepared the students in the aspects of lexis, sentence building, paragraph construction, essay coherence and rhetorical modes, which are the basic skills needed to write a research paper in English. The following chapters are designed mainly to shape the students to understand the structural layout and logic of argumentation/expression.

Before moving on to the following chapters, let's talk about a few things.

4.2 SCI, SCI paper and CNKI

SCI, Science Citation Index, compiled by the Institute for Scientific Information (ISI), is a list of scientific texts from all over the world. For each scientific paper, it has information about the author, the title, the subject, etc. All this information is taken from thousands of scientific journals.

SCI papers refer to papers included in SCI. Chinese people have a vague concept of SCI papers. A small number of people mistakenly think SCI is a journal.

SCI (Science Citation Index), EI (Engineering Index) and ISTP (Science Conference Catalogue Index) are three famous scientific literature retrieval systems in the world. They are internationally recognized as the main retrieval tools for scientific statistics and evaluation, among which SCI is the most important.

Currently, SCI publishes journals in print and CD-ROM formats, as well as online databases, and now also publishes online Web databases, covering biological and environmental sciences, medicine and life sciences, engineering technology and applied science, physics and chemistry, behavioral science and other more than 100 disciplines. Every year, more than 600,000 new articles are reported, involving 9 million citations.

There are four indexes in SCI: citation index, journal source index, subject-word index and institution index(引文索引/期刊源索引/主题词索引/机构索引). It can be retrieved over the Internet. To find SCI journals, use the following website: http://ip-science. thomsonreuters. com/mjl/.

4.2.1   Impact factors of SCI papers

The selected SCI journals are based on the literature analysis method, namely the scientific citation analysis method. In this analysis, the citation frequency of journal papers is used as the evaluation index, and the higher the citation frequency is, the greater the influence of the journal will be.

The impact factor of a journal is the total number of citations of papers published in a journal within a given period (usually the first two years) divided by the total number of papers in that journal during that period. Generally speaking, the impact factor is published in June of each year. The impact factor is not the impact factor of the year, but the impact factor of the previous year.

4.2.2   Basic requirements for SCI papers

- **Clear**: Clear thinking, Clear concept, Clear hierarchy and Clear expression.
- **Complete**: Complete content and structure.
- **Correct**: Correct scientific content, Correct data (reliable data), Correct language (Correct grammar).
- **Concise**: a treatise that clarifies scientific meaning and uses quantitative methods.

4.2.3　Understanding and thinking of SCI

From the perspective of SCI's strict selection principle and strict expert evaluation system, it has certain objectivity and could reflect the level and quality of papers in a more realistic way.

However, SCI was originally intended as a powerful document retrieval tool. Different from conventional way by subject or classification retrieval literature practice, SCI sets up a unique "citation index", a piece of literature as a search term. In this way, the context of a research project and its relevant research literature could be found quickly by collecting the cited references and following up the cited situation after publication.

Though SCI is an objective evaluation tool, it can only be used as one of the perspectives in the evaluation work, and cannot represent all the evaluated objects. Therefore, the impact factor should not be used as the only basis to evaluate the journal level, but only as one of the reference indicators.

4.2.4　Understanding CNKI

CNKI has built the most comprehensive system of China academic knowledge resources, which collected over 90% of China knowledge resources, comprehensive coverage of journals, dissertations, newspapers, proceedings, reference works, encyclopedia, patents, standards, S & T achievements and laws & regulations.

4.3　Academic research paper and its textual structure elements

Academic research papers are original works written by one or a group of researchers after careful designs, experiments, observation and statistical analysis. Research papers are the researchers' authentic academic contributions which contain their own academic views and creativities. Research papers are different from other types of papers such as review, translation and case report.

To explore the composition of a paper, EAP (English academic research papers or English academic papers) can be generally divided into experimental research and case study or literature research papers. Their textual structure elements normally consist of title, abstract, introduction, materials and methods, results, discussion, conclusions and references totally, which form an organic whole of English academic papers internationally. The text of the paper includes introduction, materials and methods, results, discussion and conclusions.

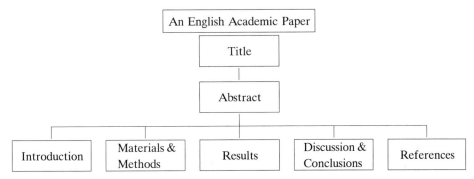

Figure 1   The textual structure elements of an English academic paper (EAP)

4.4   The basic procedure of medical research and the output process of a paper

4.4.1   Topic selection of journal papers

How are scientific papers produced? To answer this question, we must first figure out the basic procedure of medical research because writing and publishing papers is the last but also an extremely important part of the research work, which is the most effective embodiment of all the previous work.

Scientific research project/topic selection is the first step of medical research, followed by project design, research implementation, result analysis, and finally writing and publishing papers.

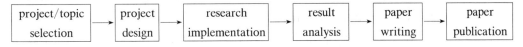

Figure 2   The basic procedure of medical research

It can be seen that this is also the basic process of quantitative scientific research.

4.4.2   The basic process of scientific research topic selection

The basic process of scientific research topic selection includes four steps. The first is to find problems in work and study. After consulting relevant literature and materials, reevaluation is conducted to analyze the feasibility and finally determine the subject or topic.

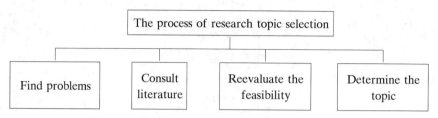

Figure 3   The basic process of research topic selection

4.4.3   Topic selection process of journal papers

The choice of a topic is a vital step in writing a research paper. Ideally a researcher should choose a topic he/she is interested in. However, it is not always an easy job to decide on an appropriate topic and establish a title accordingly, as one may be interested in many aspects of a particular topic.

A good beginning is half done, while selecting a good topic is a wise beginning of a project. A well-selected research topic should be a distilled or filtered topic that could be narrowed down enough to establish a clear focus so that the paper has a clear purpose and is not too broad or too general. Selecting a topic requires careful consideration.

To make a well-selected topic, the basic process of scientific research topic selection discussed above implies a path to follow step by step.

1. Develop a topic scope for the target problems.

Clarifying the scope of the target problem makes the topic selection path more visible and clearer. By doing so, you could take advantage of your special knowledge to make a deeper understanding of the research you have conducted or you are performing and develop one or several draft topic/topics for your paper to be written.

2. Narrow down the topic by consulting literature.

Consult and review the published SCI papers of peers in this field to confirm the research direction and specific experimental scheme you have made. In this process, you'll have some good ideas to make the topic even clearer and more perfect gradually which conforms to the project or research being done, and even in turn promote and revise the project.

Also, if no suitable topic can be found, it is time to fire up the computer and search the Internet for ideas. One of the most popular search engines, for example, is Google. A Google link for research paper topics might lead a net browser to a source that never occurred to you.

3. Focus on the topic by reevaluating the feasibility of the project.

A topic with specific focus could be developed in the process of a brief feasibility reevaluation of the project.

4. Determine the topic.

In general, after going through the three steps above, a focused topic could be determined naturally. Developing a specific focused topic will help establish a suitable title. Now you start a right way to write your research paper in English.

4.5　Ways of topic writing

4.5.1　Choose a new topic

Take your time to research for a topic. Do not settle on the first idea that pops into your head. Think it over. Ask yourself whether you would enjoy spending five weeks reading and writing about the topic. If you have doubts, keep looking until you hit on an idea that excites you. All of us are or can be excited about something. Whatever you do, do not make the mistake of choosing any old topic. Choose carelessly now, and you will pay later in boredom. Choose carefully, and you will be rewarded with the age-old excitement of research. (Winkler & Metherell, 2017)

4.5.2　Keep asking questions

One of the best ways to find a topic is to ask yourself questions about your general interests. The idea is to probe until you hit a nerve. You might begin by asking yourself some general questions. What do I want to write about? What particular subject interests me? What do I really like? If you have no immediate answer, keep asking the questions. Once you have an answer, use it to ask another, more focused question. For example, if your answer to "what do I really like?" is literature, you can then ask, "What kind of literature?" By this process, you gradually narrow down your range of writing options. It is simple, and it works. All you need is a moment of reflection.

4.5.3　Narrow down

Table 4 - 1 has listed two layers of narrowing steps. Please analyze the examples of the narrowing a researcher has to face.

Table 4 - 1　Narrowing steps

General subject	First narrowing	Second narrowing
British and American humor	British and American humor in *The Brink* and *Yes, Minister*	A contrastive study of British and American humor from the perspective of cooperative principle theory—A case study of *The Brink* and *Yes, Minister*

(Continued)

General subject	First narrowing	Second narrowing
Parallel skin	Analysis of parallel skin	Parallel skin: A vision-based dermatological analysis framework
Educational psychology	Psychological testing in schools	The thematic apperception test (TAT) and its present-day adaptations
Emergency medicine	Digital clinical pathway for emergency medicine	Development of a digital clinical pathway for emergency medicine: Lessons from usability testing and implementation failure
Chinese medicine herbs	Traditional Chinese medicine herbs in oncology clinical trials	Evaluation of traditional Chinese medicine herbs in oncology clinical trials
Clinical pharmacology	Clinical pharmacology as a medical subspecialty	Enhancing the visibility and prestige of clinical pharmacology as a medical subspecialty
Clinical teaching	Clinical teaching of oncology	Application of MDT mode in clinical teaching of oncology
Clinical genomics	Clinical genomics and precision medicine	Debutant iOS app and gene-disease complexities in clinical genomics and precision medicine
Cardiac rehabilitation interventions	Cardiac rehabilitation interventions in patients with unstable angina pectoris	The effects of cardiac rehabilitation interventions in patients with unstable angina pectoris after their incomplete revascularization

As shown in Table 4-1, the first attempt to narrow a subject usually is easier than the second, which must yield a specific topic. Use trial and error until you have a topic you like. Further narrowing may occur naturally after you are into the actual research. Remember that whatever subject you choose must be approved by your instructor.

4.6 Topics to be avoided

1. Long topics

Research topics, according to international journal articles, tend to be 10 words long or so, and a few articles have a topic of more than 20 words. Here is a case: a long topic of 23 words "Risk of poor development in young children in low-income and middle-income countries: an estimation and analysis at the global, regional, and country level."

A long topic contains many reference sources, or a bibliography, or opinion, data, or information. The solution is to narrow the topic down, focusing on the related key concept.

2. Topics of a single source

The research paper is intended to expose a researcher to the opinions of different authorities, to a variety of books, articles, and other references. If a topic is so skimpy that all the data on it come from a single source, say, a compelling biography, you are defeating the purpose of the paper. Choose only topics that are broad enough to be researched from multiple sources and are not dominated by the opinions of a single writer. (Winkler & Metherell, 2017)

3. Too technical topics

Writing about things that are technical often requires the vocabulary that might sound to your instructor like "gobbledy-gook" and be dismissed as a "snow job". Also, the skills that a research paper should teach are better learned in a paper on a general topic. Naturally, whether your paper is too technical depends on the class for which it is written. Ask your instructor. A topic like "Heisenberg's Principle of Indeterminacy as It Applies to Sub-particle Research" is fine for a physics class but a dubious choice for a class in writing. Don't stick to topics that can not be understood by any educated reader. (Winkler & Metherell, 2017)

4. Trivial topics

The definition of "trivial" is insignificant, or of no importance, such as "History of the Tennis Ball", "How to Rumor Arise in the Year Around", "Walking is Good Aerobic Exercise", and so on. Such trivial topics cannot inspire a researcher to do best writing. Therefore, trivial topics have to be avoided in research articles.

5. Hot topics

A topic that still smells of gunpowder from being hotly debated in the arena of public opinion is best avoided. There are at least two good reasons to stay away from such topics. First, it is often difficult to find unbiased sources on them; second, the information that is available usually comes from newspapers and magazines whose speculative reporting can make your documentation seem flimsy. Intellectually solid papers will reflect opinions taken from a variety of sources—books, periodicals, reference volumes, specialized indexes, and various electronic sources—which require a topic that has weathered both time and scholarly commentary.

Chapter Review

This chapter, firstly focuses on a general understanding about what an English academic paper is like. You have learnt what are SCI and SCI journals, what textual structure elements should be included in EAP, what's a basic procedure of medical research and how to select a topic.

1. In most cases, an academic paper is both argumentative and expositive.

International academic journals always have their specific requirements on paper writing especially in the following three aspects：
- the structural layout，
- logic of argumentation，
- and language expression.

2. The Science Citation Index（SCI）is a citation index originally produced by the Institute for Scientific Information（ISI）and created by Eugene Garfield. There are four indexes in SCI：
- citation index，
- journal source index，
- subject-word index，
- and institution index.

3. The textual structure of an academic research paper normally consists of 7 classic and important elements：
- title，
- abstract，
- introduction，
- materials and methods，
- results，
- discussion and conclusions，
- and references.

4. The basic process of scientific research topic selection includes four steps：
- finding problems，
- consulting relevant literature and materials，
- reevaluating and analyzing the feasibility of the topic，
- and determining the subject or topic.

Assignments

Task 1 *Answer the questions concerning information retrieval tools.*

1. In what way do people retrieve information before computers were widely used?
2. How do people often retrieve information with the help of a computer?

Task 2 *Try to write an essay covering the following three aspects：a. to answer a question；b. to discuss an issue；c. to solve a problem. The titles below may give you* *some hints.*

> • What do you think of losing weight?
> • Does government play a major role in prevention and control of major infectious diseases, such as SARS and COVID-19(新型冠状病毒性肺炎)?
> • Should humans be banned from using GMF (genetically modified food)?

Task 3   *Scan the QR code and read the titles of the SCI papers in Appendix Ⅱ, and search for at least five articles of the original text, using search engines and periodical databases.*

Task 4   *Ask your seniors for advice on how they design their subjects and choose the topics of their thesis. You'd better browse their published papers. Then discuss with your tutor about the direction of your later project. Select an article, as a reference, from Appendix Ⅱ that might be related to your conjecture topic, try to choose one or two topics, and try to write a title for it.*

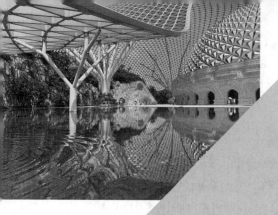

Chapter Five

Title Selection and Author-related Contents of Research Papers

Lead-in Questions

    1. What should be included in the title?

    2. What is a well-written title?

    3. What are the functions of a title?

Learning Objectives

    After learning this unit, you will be able to:

    1. identify the choice of a journal topic;

    2. know how to give your paper or study a suitable title;

    3. select good topics;

    4. correctly write author(s), corresponding author(s), their affiliated institutions and contact information.

✓参考答案
✓课件申请
✓学术资源

5.1　The function and elements of a title

The most important part of academic English paper or thesis writing is the title，which is a significant mark that distinguishes one paper from other papers. The title of a paper provides the readers with the most essential information about the whole paper. It can also be said to be the punchline of the thesis because it influences the first impression of the paper，so that readers can judge the value of the paper and its relevance to their own research，and decide whether to continue reading the paper and whether it can be retrieved.

It is a rather subjective question to clarify the function of the title because the answer will be different for different fields and for different audiences. For a hypothesis testing paper，the function of the title is to express either the topic or the message of a paper through the independent variable and the dependent variable（自变量和因变量）used in the passage. As for a medical or biomedical paper，it could be hypothetic or descriptive. Its title also has two functions：to identify both the main topic and the message of the paper and to attract readers. Generally，a title has the following functions：

　　1）to show the most important achievement(s)/results in the research，

　　2）to convey key information for the readers of the relevant field，

　　3）to indicate both the specific study and the general research field，

　　4）to illustrate the unique research methodology，

　　5）to report the location，period of time，and subjects/populations of the experiment，

　　6）to highlight the significant purpose of the work，

　　7）and to manifest the original nature of the paper.

Based on the general functions of a title，it is reasonable to infer that the main elements of a title are related to research purpose，research subject/population，research location，research materials and methods，research results and conclusions. It is a conventional rule and good idea to take these relevant elements into serious consideration when writing a well-constructed and fascinating title for a research paper. However，what kinds of elements should be included in the title actually depends on the essential point in a particular research that the writer(s) want(s) to tell the readers.

［Sample 1］

Childhood vaccines and antibiotic use in low- and middle-income countries（Lewnard et al.，2020）

[Sample 2]

Two phase 3 trials of inclisiran in patients with elevated LDL cholesterol (Ray et al., 2020)

[Analysis]

In these two samples, many relevant elements are included: the population, materials, location, method, so as to set the minimum and maximum scope of effect for the study and to generalize the population as broadly as possible within the constraints of the study.

Briefly, the title provides a distilled description of the complete article and should include information that, along with the abstract, will make electronic retrieval of the article sensitive and specific.

5.2　The main points of a title

Generally, many of the related essential factors like the specific research field, research purpose, subjects and material, are included in a title. Sometimes important research methods or other crucial factors are contained in a title. It is also proposed that final conclusion be presented in the title. Normally, there are several main points that should be noted in drawing up a title.

1) Core issues of study. That is: what problem is the research trying to solve.

[Samples 3—4]

- Inclisiran in patients at high cardiovascular risk with elevated LDL cholesterol
- Childhood vaccines and antibiotic use in low- and middle-income countries

2) Main results of the study. That is: what the most significant result of the study was.

[Samples 5—6]

- A national experiment reveals where a growth mindset improves achievement
- Diarrhoeal disease in children due to contaminated food

3) The unique material or research methodology. That is: what kind of specific materials or magnificent methods was used or created in a study?

[Samples 7—8]

- Reducing deaths from diarrhoea through spoken rehydration therapy.
- Use of quantitative molecular diagnostic methods to identify causes of diarrhoea in children: a reanalysis of the GEMS case-control study.

4) Main conclusions of the study. That is: what are the conclusions drawn from

the research results?

[**Samples 9—10**]

- Global increase and geographic convergence are in antibiotic consumption between 2000 and 2015.

- Antibiotic treatment of diarrhoea is associated with decreased time to the next diarrhoea episode among young children in Vellore, India.

5.3   The features of a title and title page

5.3.1   Four features

Based on the analysis of some international medical journals such as *Lancet*, *Nature*, *SCI Rep*, *NEJM*, and *JVI*, four common features of paper titles are identified, in spite of the characteristics of paper titles in different journals.

First, paper titles are chiefly composed of three elements: subject, objective, and methodology. Second, subtitles are mostly used in journal articles, such as "Persistence of Zika Virus in Body Fluids—Final Report" (*NEJM*, 2018). Third, many of them are in forms of noun phrases rather than sentences. Last, the average length of article titles is about 10 words. Generally speaking, good titles share the features of being concise, informative, and compliant with journal formal requirements, such as "Epidemiology of Acute Kidney Injury in Critically Ill Children and Yong Adults" from *The New England Journal of Medicine* (*NEJM*, 2017). These merits of titles will also greatly promote the acceptance of related papers, and influence the peer review and efficient citation.

5.3.2   Title pages

Most journals require a title page (cover page) in submission package which states general information about an article and its authors and usually includes the article title, author information, any disclaimers, sources of support, word count, and sometimes the number of tables and figures (mostly, as the LEGEND presented at the end of the paper).

When editors of SCI journals receive letters from authors, the first focus of attention is the title page of the manuscript because generally in the title page, the editor can roughly understand some information related to the content of the manuscript, and then make a preliminary judgment on the manuscript. So how exactly should SCI titles be written? Its contents generally include:

5.3.2.1 Article title

Accurate, concise and informative titles make deep first impression on editors and reviewers. An article title is a must.

5.3.2.2 Author information

The author's name with highest academic degree(s) and institutional affiliations where the work should be attributed should be specified, and the title page should also list the corresponding authors' (通讯作者的) telephone and fax numbers and e-mail addresses.

5.3.2.3 Disclaimers

A disclaimer is an author's statement that the views expressed in the submitted paper are his or her own and not an official position of the institution or funder.

5.3.2.4 Source(s) of support

The source(s) of support include grants, equipment, drugs, and/or other support that facilitated conduct of the work described in the paper or the writing of the paper itself. They are usually identified by:

- This study/work/research/project was supported/funded/granted/sponsored by ...
- Study/Work/Research/Project supported/funded/granted/sponsored by ...
- Supported/Funded/Granted/Sponsored by ...
- Source of funding;
- Grant sponsor.

5.3.2.5 Word count

A word count for the paper's text, excluding its abstract, acknowledgments, tables, figure legends, and references, allows editors and reviewers to assess whether the information contained in the paper warrants the paper's length, and whether the submitted manuscript fits within the journal's formats and word limits. A separate word count for the abstract is useful for the same reason.

5.3.2.6 A short running head or title

When submitting an article, journals or magazines often require running head/title. It is a short title of an article, which is usually shorter than the title and less than 40—50 English characters(字符) (not words but characters, including spaces).

5.3.2.7 Number of figures and tables

Some submission systems require specification of the number of figures and tables before uploading the relevant files. These numbers allow editorial staff and reviewers to confirm that all figures and tables were actually included with the manuscript and, because tables and figures occupy space, to assess if the information provided by the figures and tables warrants the paper's length and if the manuscript fits within the journal's space limits.

5.3.2.8 Conflict of interest declaration

Conflict of interest information for each author needs to be part of the manuscript; each journal should develop standards with regard to the form the information should take and where it will be posted. Editors may also require conflict of interest declarations on the manuscript title page. The author(s) should truthfully explain "Conflict of Interest" so as to avoid unnecessary disputes and provide references for editors to make decisions.

[**Sample 11 Title page**]

Maternal Cytomegalovirus Seroprevalence and Congenital Infection Prevalence and Its Clinical Manifestations in China

Running title: CMV Seroprevalence and Congenital Infection

Shiwen Wang* , Tongzhan Wang* , Wenqiang Zhang* , Xiaolin Liu* ,
Xiaofang Wang, Haiyan Wang, Xiaozhou He, Shunxian Zhang, Shuhui Xu,
Yang Yu, Xingbing Jia, Lijun Wang, Aiqiang Xu, Wei Ma, Minal Amin,
Stephanie R. Bialek, Sheila Dollard, Chengbin Wang

National Institute for Viral Disease Control and Prevention, Chinese Center for Disease Control and Prevention, Beijing, China (S Wang MD PhD, X Wang MD PhD, X He MD, S Zhang MD)

Shandong Provincial Key Laboratory for Infectious Disease Control and Prevention, Shandong Provincial Center for Disease Control and Prevention, Jinan, Shandong, China (T Wang MD, W Zhang MD PhD, X Liu MD, H Wang MD, A Xu MD PhD)

Jinan Municipal Center for Disease Control and Prevention, Jinan, Shandong, China (S Xu MD)

Weihai Municipal Center for Disease Control and Prevention, Weihai, Shandong, China (Y Yu MD)

Pingyin County Center for Disease Control and Prevention, Pingyin, Shandong, China (X Jia MD)

Wendeng County Center for Disease Control and Prevention, Wendeng, Shandong, China

（L Wang MD）

School of Public Health，Shandong University，Jinan，Shandong，China（W Ma MD PhD）

Centers for Disease Control and Prevention，Atlanta，Georgia，USA（M Amin MPH，S R Bialek MD，S Dollard PhD，C Wang MD PhD）

* Joint first authors

Correspondence to：Aiqiang Xu，MD，PhD，Shandong Provincial Center for Disease Control and Prevention，16992 Jingshi Road，Jinan，Shandong，250014，China，Email：axuepi@163.com，or Chengbin Wang，MD，PhD，Centers for Disease Control and Prevention，1600 Clifton Rd MS A‑34，Atlanta，Georgia，30333，USA，Email：cwang1@cdc.gov.

Word counts：XXX in abstract，XXX in text（excluding 1 figure，3 tables and XXX references）

Key Words：Cytomegalovirus，Seroprevalence，Congenital Infection

Financial Disclosure：The authors have no conflicts of interest to disclose

Funding：This study was supported by a cooperative agreement between the U. S. and China CDC，and by the Taishan Scholar Program of Shandong Provincial CDC.

Disclaimer：The findings and conclusions in this report are those of the authors and do not necessarily represent the official position of the Centers for Disease Control and Prevention.

5.4 Principles of a good title

A well-written title can function as the brand of a paper to attract editors, reviewers and readers from the very first glance，and be retrieved easily from electronic databases. Generally speaking，a well-written title should be accurate, consistent，informative and concise.

5.4.1 Accurate and consistent

An accurate title should precisely reflect the most important messages of the article by key words. The most important thing is to use the same keywords in the title as in the paper.

For a hypothesis-testing paper，find out whether your title is accurate by comparing it with the question and answer. The independent variable，the dependent variable，the animal or population，the material，the condition（if necessary），the experimental approach（if necessary），and the message（if stated）should be the same in the title as in the question and answer stated in the introduction，discussion and abstract.

[Sample 12]

Title: Neutrophil-Induced Injury of Epithelial Cells in the Pulmonary Alveoli of Rats

Questions: To determine whether the <u>injury</u> of <u>epithelial cells in the pulmonary alveoli</u> that occurs in many inflammatory conditions is <u>induced</u> in part by stimulated <u>neutrophils</u>, we exposed monolayers of purified alveolar epithelial cells from <u>rats</u> to stimulated human neutrophils and measured cytotoxicity using a ^{51}Cr-release assay.

[Analysis]

We conclude that stimulated <u>neutrophils induce injury in epithelial cells in the pulmonary alveoli</u>.

For a descriptive paper, the terms used for the structure and the function in the title should be the same as those in the message (or the message and the implication) stated in the introduction and the discussion.

[Sample 13]

Title: ARC, an Inhibitor of Apoptosis Expressed in Skeletal Muscle and Heart that Interacts Selectively with Caspases

Introduction: We have identified and characterized a human cDNA encoding an apoptosis repressor with a CARD (ARC) that is expressed in skeletal muscle and heart. ARC interacts selectively with caspases and functions as an inhibitor of apoptosis.

[Analysis]

For a method paper, the name of the method, its purpose, and the animal or population (if any) should be the same in the title as in the sections of introduction, discussion, and abstract.

[Sample 14]

Title: A Method for Purifying the Glycoprotein IIb-IIIa Complex in Platelet Membrane

Abstract: We have developed a method for the rapid purification of the glycoprotein IIb-IIIa complex in platelet membrane.

5.4.2 Concise

Short titles have more impact than long titles do, so make your title as short as possible without sacrificing accuracy and completeness. That is, to make the title concise. Some journals require a short title, usually with no more than 40 characters (including letters and spaces) on the title page or as a separate entry in an electronic submission system. Electronic submission systems may restrict the number of characters in the title. Whatever the journal's limit is, keep in mind that the aim is not to fill the space allowed. The aim is to convey the topic or the message of your paper accurately, completely, specifically, and unambiguously. If you can devise a short title that fulfills these criteria, do so. Phrases (such as noun phrases and gerunds) are often preferred to achieve conciseness. It is also advisable to avoid using "decorative" or "empty" expressions such as "A report on", "Observations on", "Some thought on", and "A research of."

Two ways to make title concise are by omitting unnecessary words and by compacting the necessary words as tightly as possible.

5.4.2.1 Omitting unnecessary words

[Sample 15]

Pharmacokinetic Studies of the Disposition of Acetaminophen in the Sheep Maternal-Placental-Fetal Unit

[Analysis]

Here "Pharmacokinetic Studies of" is regarded as nonspecific opening and should be omitted.

Revision: Disposition of Acetaminophen in the Sheep Maternal-Placental-Fetal Unit

[Sample 16]

Alterations Induced by Administration of Chlorphentermine in Phospholipids and Proteins in Alveolar Surfactant

Revision A: Alterations Induced by Chlorphentermine in Phospholipids and Proteins in Alveolar Surfactant

Revision B: Chlorphentermine-Induced Alterations in Phospholipids and Proteins in Alveolar Surfactant

5.4.2.2 Compacting necessary words

Three compacting techniques can be used to shorten titles: category terms, adjectives to express a message and noun clusters.

Category terms: One important compacting technique is to use a category term instead of details. As the following example shows, it has replaced the specific tissues with a category term, which avoids the danger of giving trees but not the forest.

[Sample 17]

Electron Microscopic Demonstration of Lysosomal Inclusion Bodies in Lung, Liver, Lymph Nodes, and Blood Leukocytes of Patients with Amiodarone-Induced Pulmonary Toxicity

Revision: Electron Microscopic Demonstration of Lysosomal Inclusion Bodies in Extrapulmonary Tissues of Patients with Amiodarone-Induced Pulmonary Toxicity

[**Analysis**]

By substituting the category term"Extrapulmonary Tissues" for liver, lymph nodes, and blood leukocytes and omitting "lung", we get the forest.

An adjective can be used instead of a noun followed by a preposition to express a message, as in the following example, where "reduced" is used instead of "reduction in."

[**Sample 18**]

Reduction in Metabolic Rate during Radio-Frequency Irradiation in Rats

Revision: Reduced Metabolic Rate during Radio-Frequency Irradiation in Rats

Noun clusters. Noun clusters sometimes can be used instead of prepositional phrases. But this technique must be used carefully to avoid creating an ambiguous title.

[**Sample 19**]

Renal Mechanism of Action of Atrial Natriuretic Factor in Rats

Revision: Renal Mechanism of Action of Rat Atrial Natriuretic Factor

5.4.3 Informative

As a condensed reflection of the paper, the title should provide enough information for the readers to know what to expect when they finish reading the whole paper. Select the most important information for the title. Keep in mind that, just as the abstract cannot replace the paper, the title cannot replace the abstract. Announcing the main information of the paper is stronger than trying to fit all the information into the title.

5.5   The structure of a title

A title is usually a noun/gerund phrase, a sentence, or even a combination of a phrase and a sentence. Prepositional phrase is often used as an effective and skillful means to modify or link other phrases in a title.

Though different written forms are required by different individual journals, a title may contain two or three sections, to emphasize two or three aspects of a research. Logically, they may be general-specific in content, or in some other relationship. In terms of message-structure, titles could be classified into three forms.

5.5.1 Topic phrase titles

A topic title is a phrase that identifies the topic of the paper. It answers the question: "What is the paper about?" A topic phrase title may be a noun phrase or a gerund phrase. For example:

1. Noun phrase
- Alcohol Use, Myocardial Infarction, Sudden Cardiac Death, and Hypertension Surgery for Infective Endocarditis
- Physician Clinical Performance Assessment: Prospects and Barriers
- An Ecological and Digital Epidemiology Analysis on the Role of Human Behavior on the 2014 Chikungunya Outbreak in Martinique

2. Gerund phrase
- Controlling Rectal Cancer
- Engaging Medical Students in the Feedback Process
- Explaining Insurance-related and Racial Disparities in the Surgical Management of Patients with Acute Appendictis

So, how exactly should SCI titles be well written or well structured? Firstly, let's observe the following three title samples and tell which one of them is a well-organized title.

[**Sample 20**]

The Relationship of Eating Kelp, the Prevention for Thyromegaly (甲状腺肿) and Adults

[**Sample 21**]

The Relationship between Eating Kelp and Prevention for Thyromegaly in Adults

[**Sample 22**]

The Effect of Eating Kelp for Prevention of Thyromegaly in Adults

[**Analysis**]

It can be seen that there involved two concepts in forms of noun phrase: eating kelp, prevention for thyromegaly. It seems reasonable and possible for the hypothesis of this study to be verified that eating kelp helps prevent people from suffering thyromegaly. However, the topic of this paper is neither about eating kelp (independent variable) nor thyromegaly (dependent variable), nor adults (population), but about the relationships between these three things.

Sample 20 is a noun phrase and looks like a topic phrase title. However, it could not implement the function of a title because the relationship between these three concepts has been explained too vague and confusing for the readers to differentiate between the three concepts within the relationship.

As for Sample 21, the population "adult" generalizes the population within the constraints of the study and the three concepts (independent variable, dependent variable and population) are clearly expressed. However, just as in Sample 20, the noun phrase "relationship" is not a proper phrase to express or present a cause and effect. Instead, Sample 22 could be a good title because it expresses the topic of the paper properly and the function of each concept involved is expressed properly.

In these two samples, many relevant elements are included: the population, materials, location, method, so as to set the minimum and maximum scope of effect for the study and to generalize the population as broad as possible within the constraints of the study.

Briefly, the title provides a distilled description of the complete article and should include information that, along with the abstract, will make electronic retrieval of the article sensitive and specific.

5.5.2   Message phrase titles

"What is the main discovery/result about the research?" is the question that a message phrase title should answer. Noun phrase and gerund phrase are also commonly used to express a message title; however, the specific discovery/result must be presented. For example, if we change the topic phrase title "The Effect of Eating Kelp for Prevention of Thyromegaly in Adults" into a message phrase title, three possible research results would create three titles respectively:

[**Sample 23**]
The Increased Incidence of Thyromegaly by Eating Kelp in Adults
[**Sample 24**]
The Decreased Incidence of Thyromegaly by Eating Kelp in Adults
[**Sample 25**]
No Effect on the Incidence of Thyromegaly by Eating Kelp in Adults

[**Analysis**]
In these three message titles above, followed the dependent variable (Incidence of Thyromegaly) are the independent variable (Eating Kelp) and the population (Adults), both of which are placed in propositional phrases. Most importantly, the dependent variable is modified by past participle (Increased and Decreased) and common negation (No) respectively so that the three message titles are created, reflecting three different experimental results.

5.5.3   Message sentence titles

In terms of grammatical structure, a message sentence title is written in the form of a sentence or even a combination of phrases and sentences. For example:
1. Sentence titles
- Human hR24L gene is involved in DNA excision repair and recombination repair.
- When should patients with heterozygous familial hypercholesterolemia be treated?

2. Combination

- Outpatient Thyroidectomy: Is It a Safe and Reasonable Option?
- Unsolved Issue: Do Drinkers Have Less Coronary Heart Disease?

In a message sentence title, the independent variable serves as the subject of a sentence and dependent as the object of the sentence; while, the verb of the sentence makes a summarized description of trend in results and the verb must be used in the present simple tense because it is a truth claim instead of a description of the result. Samples 26, 27 and 28 could help us understand the writing of message sentence titles easily.

[Sample 26]

Eating Kelp Increases the Incidence of Thyromegaly in Adults

[Sample 27]

Eating Kelp Decreases the Incidence of Thyromegaly in Adults

[Sample 28]

Eating Kelp Has No Effect on the Incidence of Thyromegaly in Adults

5.6 Some suggestions on writing a good title

1. Review and study articles published in journals that are similar to your research topic.

If you are not sure how to write a title for your article, you'd better check out journal articles on similar topics first and write your title in the same format. If you're also unsure how to use specialized vocabulary, look at articles with similar content and use the same keywords to write your title. Remember not to copy the title of other research papers.

2. The format of the topic and the number of words should conform to the requirements of the journal.

As many journals have special requirements on the format and number of article titles, it is quite necessary for us to carefully read the "Information for Authors", and avoid exceeding the word limit.

3. SCI paper titles should be accurate and original.

SCI paper titles should be accurate and original, highlighting the most important and original research findings.

4. Ensure that the title of your paper could be retrieved easily.

In order to make the title of SCI paper more searchable, the title should be written with strict and standard keywords.

5. Write a draft of a title first and make it perfect gradually.

It is a good idea to write a draft of a title at the beginning of paper writing. In the process of writing, when you have a good idea, you can revise the original title and make it perfect gradually. Sometimes, it's only in the writing process that certain nuances of meaning become clearer and give you the inspiration to write a good title.

5.7   Author, affiliation and contact information

Authors and their affiliated institutions, linked by superscript numbers or ranked by the importance of their contribution, should be listed on the opening page of the manuscript.

The e-mail, correspondence address and other contact information of the corresponding author will be published together with the paper on the opening page of the manuscript, so that other international counterparts engaged in relevant research can contact him after the paper is published.

Closely related to the authorship, the involved author's affiliations also appear, such as universities, institutes and hospitals, etc. Attention should be paid to the accuracy of the name of the involved affiliations when translated into English. For those internationally renowned institutes, their English translated names should adopt the long-used version that is generally accepted by the international academic community, so that peers can use the affiliations for literature retrieval.

[Sample 29—*Nature*]

Early prediction of circulatory failure in the intensive care unit using machine learning

Stephanie L. Hyland[1,2,3,4,10], Martin Faltys[5,10], Matthias Hüser[1,4,10], Xinrui Lyu[1,4,10], Thomas Gumbsch[6,7,10], Cristóbal Esteban[1,4], Christian Bock[6,7], Max Horn[6,7], Michael Moor[6,7], Bastian Rieck[6,7], Marc Zimmermann1, Dean Bodenham[6,7], Karsten Borgwardt[6,7,11], Gunnar Rätsch[1,2,3,4,7,8,11] and Tobias M. Merz[5,9,11]

[1]Department of Computer Science, ETH Zürich, Zürich, Switzerland. [2]Computational Biology Program, Memorial Sloan Kettering Cancer Center, New York, NY, USA. [3]Tri-Institutional PhD Program in Computational Biology and Medicine, Weill Cornell Medicine, New York, NY, USA. [4]Medical Informatics Unit, Zürich University Hospital, Zürich, Switzerland. [5]Department of Intensive Care Medicine, University Hospital, University of Bern, Bern, Switzerland. [6]Department of Biosystems Science and Engineering, ETH Zürich, Basel, Switzerland. [7]Swiss Institute for Bioinformatics, Lausanne, Switzerland. [8]Department of Biology, ETH Zürich, Zürich, Switzerland. [9]Cardiovascular Intensive Care Unit, Auckland City Hospital, Auckland, New Zealand. [10] These authors contributed equally: Stephanie L. Hyland, Martin Faltys, Matthias Hüser, Xinrui Lyu, Thomas

Gumbsch. [11] These authors jointly supervised this work: Karsten Borgwardt, Gunnar Rätsch, Tobias M. Merz. e-mail: karsten. borgwardt@bsse. ethz. ch; gunnar. raetsch@inf. ethz. ch; tobiasm@adhb. govt. nz

[**Analysis**]

Sample 29 is an excerpt from *Nature*. A title page of *Nature* should include:

- manuscript title,
- each author's name and affiliation/institution,
- contact information for corresponding authors.

In Sample 29, the authors of the paper are listed just beneath the title with Stephanie L. Hyland as the first author. The last three of the authors (Tobias M. Merz, Gunnar Rätsch and Karsten Borgwardt) are equally contributed co-corresponding authors. According to each author's linked superscript numbers, the authors' affiliated institutions are listed on the opening page of the manuscript, especially with the emails of three corresponding authors.

The authors of SCI papers should be the main accomplisher of the research reported in the papers and should participate in the process of paper writing. Chinese authors should pay attention to the British and American custom when publishing SCI papers, i. e. putting authors' first name first and last name last (uppercasing the first letter of the first name and last name respectively). At the same time, when publishing SCI papers, pay attention to the requirements of the contributing journals. The first and last name format must be unified and consistent, so as to facilitate literature retrieval by peers and understand your research comprehensively and systematically.

Among all the authors, the first author and corresponding author are the biggest contributors. The first author is usually the subject implementer, that is, the fulfiller of the main experimental tasks and the author of the paper. The corresponding author is responsible for ensuring that the descriptions are accurate, and usually the chief person in charge of the research, determining the idea of the project or research, providing experimental funds and reviewing the paper. Some SCI journals allow authors with equivalent contributions to be co-first authors or co-corresponding authors, for example, "Drs. Ray and Wright contributed equally to this article."

The authors of SCI papers should be listed in the order of first author, other authors and corresponding authors. Other authors, often more than one, should be ranked in descending importance according to their degree of contribution. The ranking of authors is related to recognition of the importance of their work and must be agreed between the first author and the corresponding author and approved by other authors.

[**Sample 30—*N Engl J Med***]

Observational Study of Hydroxychloroquine in Hospitalized Patients with COVID-19

Joshua Geleris, M. D. , Yifei Sun, Ph. D. , Jonathan Platt, Ph. D. , Jason Zucker, M. D. , Matthew Baldwin, M. D. , George Hripcsak, M. D. , Angelena Labella, M. D. , Daniel K. Manson, M. D. , Christine Kubin, Pharm. D. , R. Graham Barr, M. D. , Dr. P. H. , Magdalena E. Sobieszczyk, M. D. , M. P. H. , and Neil W. Schluger, M. D.

From the Divisions of General Medicine, Infectious Diseases, and Pulmonary, Allergy, and Critical Care Medicine, Department of Medicine (J. G. , J. Z. , M. B. , A. L. , D. K. M. , C. K. , R. G. B. , M. E. S. , N. W. S.), the Departments of Biostatistics (Y. S.) and Epidemiology (J. P. , R. G. B. , N. W. S.), Mailman School of Public Health, and the Department of Biomedical Informatics (G. H.), Vagelos College of Physicians and Surgeons, Columbia University, and New York—Presbyterian Hospital—Columbia University Irving Medical Center (J. G. , J. Z. , M. B. , A. L. , D. K. M. , C. K. , R. G. B. , M. E. S. , N. W. S.) — all in New York. Address reprint requests to Dr. Schluger at the Division of Pulmonary, Allergy, and Critical Care Medicine, Columbia University Irving Medical Center, PH-8 E. , Rm. 101, 622 W. 168th St. , New York, NY 10032, or at ns311@cumc. columbia. edu.

[**Analysis**]

A title page of *N Engl J Med* should include:

- manuscript title,
- each author's name, highest degree, and affiliation/institution,
- contact information for the corresponding author.

In Sample 30, Dr. Geleris is the first author. Dr. Schluger is the corresponding author and his correspondence address and e-mail are included at the end of the list of the authors' affiliation.

Chapter Review

A good title of a research paper provides a distilled description of the complete article and should include information that, along with the abstract, will make electronic retrieval of the article sensitive and specific.

Based on the functions and main elements of a title, in this chapter, we have also discussed the main points, common principles, features and structure of a good title, and title page in international medical journals. Finally, some ways of writing a good title are suggested.

1. It is a conventional rule and good idea to take some relevant elements of a title into consideration seriously when writing a well-constructed and fascinating

title for a research paper.
- Easy to understand
- Accurate promise of the paper's content
- Specifying the scope of the study
- No use of unexplained abbreviations unless they are widely accepted by the target journal's audience (e.g. HIV, AIDS, DNA, RNA, IQ)
- Simple, short, concise
- 10 to 12 words long
- Interesting
- Stating the subject of the article, sometimes the conclusion
- Nondeclarative
- Indicating the study design
- Eye-catching
- Beginning with a key word
- Grammatically correct
- Worded appropriately for the target journal's audience

2. There are several main points that should be noted in drawing up a title.
- Core issues of the study to answer the question: what problem is the research trying to solve?
- Main results of the study to answer the question: what was the most significant result of the study?
- Sometimes, the unique material or research methodology.
- Main conclusions of the study concerning what are the conclusions drawn from the research.

3. Three forms of title structure:
- A topic title: about the question "What is the paper about?"
- A message title: about "What is the main discovery/result about the research?"
- A message sentence title: written in the form of sentence or even a combination of phrase and sentence.

Assignments

Task 1   *Search the journals in your specialty to find some papers with titles of the following types.*

Noun Phrases

_____

_____

Gerunds

_____

_____

Sentences

_____

_____

Combination

_____

_____

Task 2   *Rewrite the following titles to make them concise and clear.*

1. A study of two cases of primary sclerosing cholangitis
2. Studies on the pathogenesis of refractory anemia
3. Investigation of pathology of noncirrhotic portal fibrosis
4. Discussion on cause of anemia in malaria
5. Evaluation of etiology of liver disease in renal-transplant patients
6. On histologic classification of thyroid cancer

Task 3   *Mark out the steps you think are useful for writing a title.*

1. Write a draft of a title at the beginning of the paper writing and make it perfect gradually in the process of writing.
2. Rewrite the title after the paper is finished since you have got a very clear idea about the paper then.

3. Decide what kind of structural title you are going to write according to the general topic structure of the journal you are submitting to.

4. Study the linguistic features of titles in the journal that you are going to submit your paper to.

5. Correctly express three concepts: the independent variables, dependent variables and population.

6. Pick out the most informative words.

7. Revise the title to maximize the meaningful content within an appropriate length.

8. Link all the phrases with proper linking devices.

9. Use noun phrases or gerunds to present dependent variables.

10. Include the core study issue, main study result and main conclusion exactly in the title.

11. Review and study articles published in journals that are similar to your research topic.

12. Make sure that the title of your paper could be retrieved easily.

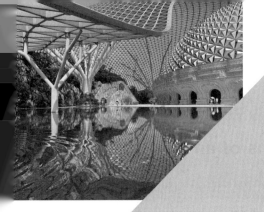

Chapter Six

Abstract Writing

Lead-in Questions

1. Should you write your abstract before or after finishing the body of your paper?

2. Have you ever read some abstracts in your study field?

3. Have you ever read abstracts to consult relevant reference in your study field?

4. Are there any uniformed standards for writing medical abstract?

Learning Objectives

After learning this chapter, you will be able to:

1. understand function, characteristics and processing of abstract writing,

2. and understand the five "moves" included in the abstract and try to get some writing practice.

✓参考答案
✓课件申请
✓学术资源

6.1　An overview and functions of an abstract

The abstract is the first section of an experimental research paper, served as the point of entry, coming after the title and before the section of introduction. Besides the title, an abstract is the most frequently read part of a research paper. It is a part of a published paper that biomedical and clinical researchers can read for free when they use PubMed, an online search engine, for literature retrieval.

The abstract provides the readers with a brief preview of the study based on information from the other sections of the paper. It is the epitome, refinement and summary of scientific research works. The abstract can be called a miniature version of an article. APA (American Psychological Association) defines abstract as:

A brief, comprehensive summary of the contents of the article; it allows readers to survey the contents of an article quickly, and like a title, it enables abstracting and information services to index and retrieve articles.

This definition also indicates that the abstract is used as an important measure for retrieving papers and for promoting the international sci-tech exchange. Generally, it is used to accomplish three important tasks:

- to help readers identify the interest of a paper,
- to outline the main points of a paper,
- and to guide the reading of a paper.

Before the paper comes in official publication, the abstract impresses the editor about the content and quality of the paper and help the editor decide whether the article is worth publishing. A well-written abstract, therefore, contributes much to the acceptance and publication of the article.

Once the article is published, the abstract will be indexed in many electronic databases, and it will help readers to locate and retrieve the article quickly and efficiently. Before reading through the paper, readers can have a general understanding of the core problems to be solved, research methods to be studied, important conclusions, etc., and get an overall impression of the work to judge the content of the paper and relevance to their research work.

Briefly speaking, an abstract plays a vital role for its author to convince the journal editor to accept and publish his/her paper first, by providing an overview and specific highlight of the paper. The other main function of an abstract is to provide specific key elements from each of the other sections of the paper, by providing its readers with a brief preview about the whole paper, and with explicit or implicit information about research background, introduction, purposes, methods, results and conclusions of the paper, upon which its readers might depend to decide whether to read the paper or not. Thus, the abstract should make sense both when read alone and when read with the paper.

6.2 Abstract identification and academic summary

To learn how to write normative abstracts, we'd better make clear what an abstract is like and what an academic summary is like because they are easily confused.

An abstract and academic summary both highlight the major points in an article or a paper and they are separated from the article. However, they are quite different from each other: an abstract is a short statement about an article designed to give a complete yet concise understanding of its research and findings while an academic summary is a brief and concise restatement of the main facts or points of an article or a book; an abstract usually appears at the beginning of the paper as the point of entry while a summary at the end of an article; an abstract is more condensed and thus shorter than a summary (normally with only one paragraph), which must contain key words (essential in a paper).

Now, read through the following two samples and try to get a general feeling or sense about their tone, writing style, linguistic features and discourse structure, etc.

[**Sample 1 Abstract**]

A national experiment reveals where a growth mindset improves achievement

Abstract: (1) A global priority for the behavioural sciences is to develop cost-effective, scalable interventions that could improve the academic outcomes of adolescents at a population level, but no such interventions have so far been evaluated in a population-generalizable sample. (2) Here we show that a short (less than one hour), online growth mindset intervention—which teaches that intellectual abilities can be developed—improved grades among lower-achieving students and increased overall enrollment to advanced mathematics courses in a nationally representative sample of students in secondary education in the United States. (3) Notably, the study identified school contexts that sustained the effects of the growth mindset intervention: the intervention changed grades when peer norms aligned with the messages of the intervention. (4) Confidence in the conclusions of this study comes from independent data collection and processing, preregistration of analyses, and corroboration of results by a blinded Bayesian analysis. (Yeager et al., 2019)

[Sample 2　Summary]

Summary：The authors in this study assessed the relationship between job performance in first-level managers (as rated by their supervisors) and their affective commitment, continuance commitment, and job satisfaction. Affective commitment is defined as an emotional attachment to the organization (Meyer, Paunonen, Gellatly, Goffin, & Jackson, 1989). Alternatively, continuance commitment is based on the costs that employees associate with leaving the organization. Job performance was assessed according to 3 dimensions (1) composite performance, according to an average on 6 specific activities, (2) overall performance, based on a subjective rating given by the immediate supervisor, and (3) promotability. The participants were 23 district managers and 65 unit managers from a large food service organization. The researchers found that affective commitment was positively related to overall performance and promotability. The correlations between continuance commitment and all 3 performance dimensions were negative and significant. What I learned from this article and these findings is that supervisor ratings of performance and promotability increase as the employees' affective commitment increases; on the other hand, supervisor ratings of performance and promotability decrease as continuance commitment increases.

[Analysis]

Both of the samples above have some similar highlights or the major points to be explained or declared, such as methods and materials, study purpose, results and conclusions. However, they are quite different in their tone, writing style, linguistic features and discourse structure, etc.

The typical abstract usually consists of five parts or moves: introduction, purpose, methods, results and conclusion. On the other hand, an academic summary typically outlines four elements relevant to the completed work: research focus, research method, results/findings, conclusion and recommendation. Sample 2 is a proper academic summary.

6.3　Moves in an abstract

There are chiefly three types of abstracts according to their functions: descriptive abstracts, evaluative abstracts and informative abstracts. When most people use the word "abstract" they are probably referring to the informative abstract. No personal feelings or thoughts are injected; the main points of the material are presented objectively. It serves as a substitute of the original and is the proper form for paper retrieving. Sci-tech/research paper abstracts, including biomedical and clinical medicine papers, are usually written in this form.

6.3.1　Five moves or key elements in the abstract

Usually, five moves or key elements are included in the abstract.

Table 6 - 1　Moves or key elements in the abstract

Move	Key elements	Functions/contents/tense
Move 1	Introduction/ Background	Introduces the background, present situation, problems, etc., usually written in the present tense.
Move 2	Purpose	States the premise, purpose, problem, task, or thesis of the research, usually written in the past tense.
Move 3	Methods	States the principles, objects, population, location, materials, technology, methods or procedures of the research, usually written in the past tense.
Move 4	Results	States the results, such as the data, effects or properties of the research, usually written in the past tense.
Move 5	Conclusions/ Implications	Gives comparison or application of the results, or raises questions, recommendations or predictions on the basis of the results, usually written in the present tense.

6.3.2　Move-reduced abstract

Abstracts should be as brief and concise as possible and the submitted abstract must fit within the journal's formats and word limits. In order to satisfy such requirement, the background information can be omitted.

The reduced abstract typically focuses on only two or three elements, with the emphasis placed on the results of the study. Information concerning the purpose and method is presented first. Then the most important results are summarized. Finally, conclusions and recommendations may be included in one or two sentences.

Moves of Information Elements in Reduced Abstract 1

- Purpose
- Methods of the study
- Results
- Conclusions and/or recommendations

Moves of Information Elements in Reduced Abstract 2

- Background/introduction
- Methods of the study
- Results
- Conclusions and/or recommendations

6.3.3　Move discourse

6.3.3.1　Move 1 and Move 2

Usually, the text of an abstract starts from Move 1 and/or Move 2. To make the abstract short, Move 1 can be omitted. There are basically four types of abstract-opening sentences (Swales & Feak, 2009).

Type 1: Start with an introduction of background information.

E. g. Anemia(贫血), which is common in the critically ill, is often treated with red-cell transfusions, which are associated with poor clinical outcomes.

Type 2: Start with a problem or a doubt, often combined with Type 1.

E. g. Very few studies ... have focused on emerging infections, generating a gap of knowledge that hampers epidemiological response planning.

E. g. Types 1 + 2: The congenital cytomegalovirus (CMV) infection is the leading viral cause of birth defects and developmental disabilities in developed countries. However, the CMV seroprevalence and congenital CMV infection are not well defined in China yet.

Type 3: Start with study purpose or objective, or study purpose and method.

E. g. To investigate the help-seeking behaviors and related factors of Chinese psychiatric inpatients with schizophrenia ... .

E. g. To determine the bacteria causing stomach troubles, biopsy specimens were taken from intact areas of antral mucosa in 100 consecutive consenting patients presenting for gastroscopy.

Type 4: Start with present research action.

E. g. We performed a pairwise epistatic interaction test using the chicken 60 K single nucleotide polymorphism (SNP) chip for the 11th generation of the Northeast Agricultural University broiler lines divergently selected for abdominal fat content.

6.3.3.2　Move 3

Lots of information should be described concisely in Move 3 which states many key-detailed points of the study methods like the principles, objects or population, data, location, materials, technology, methods or procedures of the research. This information must be refined and distilled.

E. g.

Methods: Newborns from five birthing hospitals in two counties of Shandong Province, China, were enrolled from March 2011 to October 2013. Dried blood spots (DBS) and saliva were collected from heel stick or swabs within 4 days after birth. CMV IgG was tested on DBS with ELISA for maternal seroprevalence assessment. Real time PCR was performed on saliva and DBS for viral detection of congenital CMV infection.

6.3.3.3 Move 4

Move 4 is thought to be the most important part of an abstract. In Move 4, the results of a study are summarized, usually in order of importance. There are two basic writing structures: list-to-summary type and general-to-specific type.

[**Sample 3 Move 4**]

Here, we analyze the case of a Chikungunya outbreak that occurred in Martinique in 2014. Using time series estimates from a network of sentinel practitioners covering the entire island, we first analyze the spatio-tempspoken dynamics and show that the largest city has served as the epicenter of this epidemic. We further show that the epidemic spread from there through two different propagation waves moving northwards and southwards, probably by individuals moving along the road network. We then develop a mathematical model to explore the drivers of the femoral dynamics of this mosquito-borne virus. Finally, we show that human behavior, inferred by a textual analysis of messages published on the social network Twitter, is required to explain the epidemiological dynamics over time. Overall, our results suggest that human behavior has been a key component of the outbreak propagation, and we argue that such results can lead to more efficient public health strategies specifically targeting the propagation process. (Roche et al., 2017)

[**Analysis**]

Sample 3 is a list-to-summary type of Move 4. The specific results of the study are listed one by one, then a summary of the results is presented. By the way, Sample 3 is also a good example of Moves 3 & 4 combined type.

In quantitative studies, Move 4 of the abstract tends to provide exact numbers and percentages. See the following sample of list-to-summary type of Move 4.

[**Sample 4 Move 4**]

A total of 5,020 newborns had CMV IgG tested and 4,827 were seropositive with CMV seroprevalence of 96.2% [95% confidence interval (CI):95.6%—96.7%]. Of the 10,933 newborns screened for congenital CMV infection, 75 had CMV detected with prevalence of 0.7% (95% CI: 0.5%—0.8%). Congenital CMV infection prevalence decreased along with increased maternal age (0.9%, 0.6%, and 0.3% among newborns from mothers aged 16—25 years, 26—35 years, and >35 years, respectively; $P = 0.03$), and was higher among newborns with preterm birth (1.3% vs. 0.6%, $P = 0.04$), with intrauterine growth restriction (1.8% vs. 0.7%, $P = 0.03$), and twins or triplets (2.4% vs. 0.7%, $P = 0.002$).

[Sample 5　Move 4]

(1) The models show that feedbacks between the biological and economic systems can lead to a state of persistent poverty. (2) Analyses of a wide range of specific systems under alternative assumptions show the existence of three possible regimes corresponding to a globally stable development equilibrium ... (Ngonghald，2017)

[Analysis]

Sample 5 is the type of general-to-specific. The first sentence indicates the general results of the models of the paper，while the specific findings/results are presented from the second sentence.

6.3.3.4　Move 5

In Move 5，the conclusions or implications of a study are stated directly or indirectly by giving some points like comparison or application of the results, questions，recommendations or predictions on the basis of the results. Major tendencies and significant individual or grouped results are emphasized. Whether or not Move 5 is included in an abstract depends on the research itself and the requirements or the target journal. In biomedical and clinical fields，an abstract is more likely to include Move 5，to stress the significance or applicability of the result.

[Sample 6　Move 5]

Overall，our results suggest that human behavior has been a key component of the outbreak propagation，and we argue that such results can lead to more efficient public health strategies specifically targeting the propagation process (Roche et al. , 2017).

[Sample 7　Move 5]

CONCLUSIONS：The majority of cases of XDR tuberculosis in KwaZulu-Natal，South Africa，an area with a high tuberculosis burden，were probably due to transmission rather than to inadequate treatment of MDR tuberculosis. These data suggest that control of the epidemic of drug-resistant tuberculosis requires an increased focus on interrupting transmission. (Funded by the National Institute of Allergy and Infectious Diseases and others) (Shah et al. , 2017)

6.4　Requirements for an abstract

By reading an abstract, the readers can understand the broad content, results and conclusions without needing to read the whole paper (McCormack & Slaght, 2015, p.73). However，different SCI journals have different requirements for abstract writing, which are detailed in Instructions to Authors or Guideline for Authors. The author should write his/her abstract according to the writing requirements of the journal, or modify the abstract to meet the requirements of the target journal.

6.4.1   The writing requirements of *NEJM* for abstract

NEJM details its requirements for the abstract as:

> Provide an abstract of not more than 250 words. It should consist of four paragraphs, labelled background, methods, results and conclusion. They should briefly describe, respectively, the problem being addressed in the study, how the study was performed, the salient results, and what the authors conclude from the others.

[Analysis]

It can be seen that *NEJM* requires authors to put forward structured abstracts.

6.4.2   The writing requirements of *Science* for abstract

In the Instructions to Authors, *Science* details its writing requirements for the abstract as:

> Abstracts explain to the general reader why the research was done, what was found and why the results are important. They should start with some brief BACKGROUND information: a sentence giving a broad introduction to the field comprehensible to the general reader, and then a sentence of more detailed background specific to your study. This should be followed by an explanation of OBJECTIVES/METHODS and then the RESULTS. The final sentence should outline the main CONCLUSION of the study, in terms that will be comprehensible or to all our readers. The abstract is distinct from the main body of the text. Please do not include citations or abbreviations in the Abstract. The abstract should be 125 words or less.

[Analysis]

In the Instructions to Authors of *Science*, it is suggested that *Science* usually requires non-structured abstracts.

6.4.3   The writing requirements of *Internal Medicine Journal* for abstract

Internal Medicine Journal makes the following abstract requirements in its author guideline:

> Each manuscript should carry a structured abstract of not more than 250 words presented in the following form. Background: brief statement of relevant

work or clinical situation，and hypothesis，if applicable. Aims：brief statement of the overall aim. Methods：laboratory or other techniques used，including statistical analysis. Outcome measures clearly stated. Results：statistically significant results and relevant negative data cited. Conclusions：referable to the aims of the study and may include suggestions for future action.

6.5 Formats of an abstract

Different academic journals require different abstract formats. Generally，abstracts fall into two categories：non-structured abstracts and structured abstracts.

6.5.1 Non-structured abstracts

A non-structured abstract is more traditional format. It consists of only one paragraph with about 250 words，all written in complete sentences. This abstract paragraph must be complete with itself for its readers before reading the full paper and it has no citations，no references.

The abstract could start with background（Move 1）if it is necessary for understanding the hypothesis of the paper. Otherwise，the abstract could directly start from Move 2 or Move 3.

Although a non-structured abstract has no headings，it should include all the most important information/elements of the article. The element content should be presented in the same order as the body of the paper，starting from a general introduction（Move 1，if necessary），moving on to more specific element contents（methods，materials and results），and ending with a touch on conclusions or discussion. In the course of different move-developing，signal words or phrases should be used for transition from move to move.

In spite of the traditional format，a non-structured abstract continues to be used by many SCI journals like *Science*，*Nature* and *JVI*（*Journal of Virology*），etc.

［**Sample 8 A non-structured abstract**］
DNA vaccine protection against SARS-CoV-2 in rhesus macaques（恒河猴）
（1）The global COVID-19 pandemic（COVID-19 大流行）caused by the SARS-CoV-2 virus has made the development of a vaccine a top biomedical priority.（2）In this study，we developed a series of DNA vaccine candidates expressing different forms of the SARS-CoV-2 Spike（S）protein and evaluated them in 35 rhesus macaques.（3）Vaccinated animals developed humoral and cellular immune responses，including neutralizing antibody titers comparable to those found in convalescent humans and macaques infected with SARS-CoV-

2. (4) Following vaccination, all animals were challenged with SARS-CoV-2, and the vaccine encoding the full-length S protein resulted in >3.1 and >3.7 $\log_{10}$ reductions in median viral loads in bronchoalveolar lavage and nasal mucosa, respectively, as compared with sham controls. (5) Vaccine-elicited neutralizing antibody titers correlated with protective efficacy, suggesting an immune correlate of protection. (6) These data demonstrate vaccine protection against SARS-CoV-2 in nonhuman primates. (Yu et al., 2020)

[Analysis]

This is a paper published in *Science* in 2020. It is a non-structured abstract, which is consistent with the requirements of *Science* for abstract. In the fourth sentence, the results are reported and a research method is explained, because it is a more technique-oriented paper. The following table helps us understand the writing of non-structured abstract by the sample illustration.

Table 6 - 2　The format of a non-structured abstract

Sentence	Move	Information	Signal(direct or implied)
(1)	Move 1	Broad background	
(2)	Move 1	Detailed background	In this study
(3)	Move 4	First result	Vaccinated animals developed
(4)	Moves 4 & 3	Second result and method	Following vaccination, challenged, as compared with sham controls
(5) & (6)	Move 5	Conclusion	... suggesting an immune correlate of protection, These data demonstrate ...

6.5.2　Structured abstracts

Although a large number of biomedical and medical journals are still using non-structured abstracts, the trend is that more are shifting to a structured format. Structured abstracts briefly provide the important points of the study by using subheadings. One obvious difference between a non-structured abstract and a structured one is that a structured abstract is multi-paragraph, with each paragraph under a heading.

Structured abstracts have been used by many SCI journals, such as *NEJM* (*the New England Journal of Medicine*), *Lancet*, *HIV Medicine*, *Internal Medicine Journal*, *Nuclear Medicine and Biology*, *British Journal of Surgery*. According to the recommendations of *ICMJE*, original research, systematic reviews, and meta-analyses require structured abstracts. The abstract should provide the context or background for the study and should state the study's purpose, basic procedures (selection of study participants, settings, measurements, analytical methods), main findings (giving specific effect sizes and their statistical and clinical significance, if possible), and principal conclusions. It should emphasize new and important aspects of the study or observations, note important limitations, and not overinterpret findings. Clinical trial abstracts should include items that the CONSORT group has identified as essential (*www. consort-statement. org/resources/downloads/extensions/consort-extension-for-abstracts-2008pdf/*). Funding sources should be listed separately after the abstract to facilitate proper display and indexing for search retrieval by *MEDLINE*.

Journals differ widely on the format for abstracts, including the non-structured format. Before submitting your paper, you have to read the relevant requirements specific to the target journal, and read through some previous published papers to see what headings should be included in the structured abstract of your target journal.

Take 2-3 minutes to browse through the following sample of structured abstract cited from *NEJM*. (Paz-Bailey et al., 2018)

[**Sample 9—A structured abstract**]

Persistence of Zika Virus in Body Fluids
—Final Report

BACKGROUND

To estimate the frequency and duration of detectable Zika virus (ZIKV) RNA in human body fluids, we prospectively assessed a cohort of recently infected participants in Puerto Rico.

METHODS

We evaluated samples obtained from 295 participants (including 94 men who provided semen specimens) in whom ZIKV RNA was detected on reverse-transcriptase-polymerase-chain-reaction (RT-PCR) assay in urine or blood at an enhanced arboviral clinical surveillance site. We collected serum, urine, saliva, semen, and vaginal secretions weekly for the first month and at 2, 4, and 6 months. All specimens were tested by means of RT-PCR, and serum was tested with the use of anti-ZIKV IgM enzyme-linked immunosorbent assay. Among the participants with ZIKV RNA in any specimen at week 4, collection continued every 2 weeks thereafter until all specimens tested negative. We used parametric Weibull regression models to estimate the time until the loss of ZIKV RNA detection in each body fluid and reported the findings in medians and 95th percentiles.

RESULTS

The medians and 95th percentiles for the time until the loss of ZIKV RNA detection were 15 days (95% confidence interval [CI], 14 to 17) and 41 days (95% CI, 37 to 44), respectively, in serum; 11 days (95% CI, 9 to 12) and 34 days (95% CI, 30 to 38) in urine; and 42 days (95% CI, 35 to 50) and 120 days (95% CI, 100 to 139) in semen. Less than 5% of participants had detectable ZIKV RNA in saliva or vaginal secretions.

CONCLUSIONS

The prolonged time until ZIKV RNA clearance in serum in this study may have implications for the diagnosis and prevention of ZIKV infection. In 95% of the men in this study, ZIKV RNA was cleared from semen after approximately 4 months. (Funded by the Centers for Disease Control and Prevention.)

[Analysis]

The advantage of a structured abstract is that readers can quickly find the element of the research that is relevant to their particular situation or interest. To some extent, structured abstracts will be more concise and carry more information than non-structured abstracts.

6.6   The process of abstract writing

6.6.1   The process of abstract writing

(1) Write your abstract after the paper is finished;

(2) Before submitting your paper, read the relevant requirements in the Instructions to Authors specific to the target journal to see what kind of abstract format is required;

(3) Read through some of the abstracts of previous published papers of your target journal to see what elements or headings should be included and what detailed information of each element or heading should be explained;

(4) Read your original paper carefully to get the overall picture and a deeper understanding;

(5) Sort out a clear clue to your study's main points including the move elements (background, materials and methods, results and conclusions) and their important information, then list them in the note form;

(6) Write your abstract according to the writing requirements of the target journal, with the understanding of your preparation and study work for abstract writing;

(7) Modify the abstract to meet the requirements of the target journal, using transitional words and phrases where necessary to ensure coherence;

(8) Submit your paper with a good abstract.

6.6.2   Usages of abstracts

Abstracts allow researchers to find and assess a wide range of relevant work, thus remaining in touch with the large quantity of literature in their field. In effect, they assist the wider academic community in working together on common problems or areas of interest. When searching for information, researchers use key words to find relevant information. An abstract should therefore contain key words in relation to the article or paper, for ease of retrieval.

As a student, it is very useful to read an abstract in order to find out quickly about the main idea of a text, and thus to decide whether the text is relevant to your needs. You may be expected to include abstracts at the beginning of pieces of extending writings, as well as to submit an abstract if you are going to give a presentation based on your project.

Chapter Review

This chapter is designed to consolidate the learners' understanding of research abstract writing in terms of the function of the abstract, moves included in the abstract, requirements for abstracts and formats of abstract.

1. According to Swales and Feak (2009), there are four basic types of abstract-opening sentences:

Type 1: Start with an introduction of background information;

Type 2: Start with a problem or a doubt often combined with Type 1;

Type 3: Start with study purpose or objective, or study purpose and method;

Type 4: Start with present research action.

2. Different academic journals require different abstract formats. Generally, abstracts fall into two categories:

• non-structured abstracts;

• structured abstracts.

3. Your abstract must be written according to the requirements of the target journal. Different SCI journals have different requirements for abstract writing, which are detailed in Instructions to Authors or Guideline for Authors. The author should write his/her abstract according to the writing requirements of the journal, or modify the abstract to meet the requirements of the target journal.

Assignments

Task 1 *Read at least 10 opening sentences in your own reference corpus of abstracts, and identify the opening Move-type they fall into. Is there any type you cannot classify?*

Task 2 *Discuss with your partner: Should you write your abstract before or after you finish the paper? What is your strategy for deciding what key words to identify?*

Task 3   *The following disordered sentences are taken from an abstract, entitled "Childhood Vaccines and Antibiotic Use in Low- and Middle-income Countries" (Lewnard, 2020), focusing on functional key words and context move and ignoring unfamiliar words. Rearrange these sentences into a well-organized non-structured abstract by numbering them from 1 to 7.*

_____A. Here we show that vaccines that have recently been implemented in the World Health Organization's Expanded Programme on Immunization reduce antibiotic consumption substantially among children under five years of age in LMICs.

_____B. Under current coverage levels, pneumococcal and rotavirus vaccines prevent 23. 8 million and 13. 6 million episodes of antibiotic-treated illness, respectively, among children under five years of age in LMICs each year.

_____C. Vaccines may reduce the burden of antimicrobial resistance, in part by preventing infections for which treatment often includes the use of antibiotics.

_____D. By analysing data from large-scale studies of households, we estimate that pneumococcal conjugate vaccines and live attenuated rotavirus vaccines confer 19.7% (95% confidence interval, 3. 4%—43. 4%) and 11. 4% (4. 0%—18. 6%) protection against antibiotic-treated episodes of acute respiratory infection and diarrhea, respectively, in age groups that experience the greatest disease burden attributable to the vaccine-targeted pathogens.

_____E. However, the effects of vaccination on antibiotic consumption remain poorly understood—especially in low-and middle-income countries (LMICs), where the burden of antimicrobial resistance is greatest.

_____F. This evidence supports the prioritization of vaccines within the global strategy to combat antimicrobial resistance.

_____G. Direct protection resulting from the achievement of universal coverage targets for these vaccines could prevent an additional 40. 0 million episodes of antibiotic-treated illness.

Task 4 *Write an abstract of 250 words and decide key words for the research paper below.*

Cohort study on maternal cytomegalovirus seroprevalence and prevalence and clinical manifestations of congenital infection in China

1. Introduction

Congenital cytomegalovirus (CMV) infection results from vertical transmission of CMV from mother to the fetus during pregnancy. Although any maternal infection during pregnancy, primary or nonprimary (reinfection and reactivation), can result in congenital CMV infection, the risk of vertical viral transmission is lower in nonprimary than primary maternal infections.[1] Moreover, congenital CMV infections from nonprimary maternal infection are less likely to present with symptoms at birth, and are thought to be less likely to result in long-term permanent sequelae such as hearing loss and developmental disabilities. [2] CMV infection is well documented as the leading viral cause of birth defects and developmental disabilities in developed countries[3], which typically have moderate maternal seroprevalences of 40% to 70%. [4-7] However, the epidemiology of congenital CMV infection in developing countries with very high maternal seroprevalence (>90%) is not as well understood. [8,9] With high CMV seroprevalence, congenital CMV infection is less attributable to maternal primary infection than in countries with lower maternal seroprevalence. [10,11] Moreover, the likelihood of symptomatic infection and permanent sequelae among infants with congenital infection in these populations is unknown. To investigate congenital CMV prevalence and its clinical manifestations in China, where maternal CMV seroprevalence is reported to be higher than 95%,[12] we conducted universal screening for congenital CMV infection among infants born in 2 counties of Shandong Province, China.

2. Methods

2.1 Study population and data collection

Newborn screening for congenital CMV infection was conducted from March 2011 to August 2013 in 5 birthing hospitals of Pingyin and Wendeng Counties of Shandong Province which comprised more than 80% of infants delivered in the 2 counties. Wendeng County was more populous (609 737 vs 331 712 in 2010 census) and had a higher GDP per capita (96 249 *yuan*, approximately 15 778 US dollars) than Pingyin County (44 128 *yuan*, approximately 7 234 US dollars). GDP in both of these counties was higher than the national GDP per capita (6 265 US dollars in 2012). The birthrate in Pingyin County was higher than in Wendeng County (9.5‰ vs 7.4‰).

All parents were approached in the hospital about enrolling their infants before delivery, with more than 90% of infants enrolled. Demographic information on the mothers was collected by interviews by research staff. Information on delivery and outcomes of routine clinical evaluations, including newborn hearing screening, was collected from the medical record. Newborn hearing screening was typically conducted at least 48 hours after birth and before discharge in the birthing hospitals using transiently evoked otoacoustic emissions (AccuScreen, Denmark). Infants who failed were retested within 6 weeks after birth and referred for diagnostic hearing testing within 3 months of age if they failed the rescreen.

Microcephaly was defined as head circumference exceeding 2 standard deviations below the mean according to international newborn standard values,[13] assessed for a majority of infants but not infants during the 1st year of the study. Intrauterine growth restriction (IUGR) was defined as birth weight less than the 5th percentile of the gender-specific gestational age-corrected standard reference values for Chinese infants.[14] Symptomatic congenital CMV infection was defined as presence of microcephaly, petechiae, or seizure detected through routine newborn care before discharge, along with congenital CMV infection which was identified by real-time PCR. Congenital CMV infection without any of these 3 symptoms at birth was defined as asymptomatic congenital CMV infection.

2.2　Specimen collection and laboratory testing

Specimens were collected from the enrolled infants within 4 days of birth. Dried blood spots (DBS) were collected using 903 Whatman filter paper (GE Healthcare, UK) only from infants enrolled during the first 12 months of the 30-month study period. Saliva specimens were collected from all infants enrolled in the study using a sterile polyester swab that was placed in the infant's mouth against the cheek and rotated for 10 seconds. To prevent potential contamination from breast milk, saliva specimens were collected at least 1 hour after breast feeding. Saliva specimens were frozen immediately, stored at 20 ℃ and transported on ice to the testing laboratory (wet saliva). In order to compare saliva collection methods, a 2nd saliva specimen was collected from infants enrolled during the last 12 months of the study and air dried at room temperature overnight, placed in small tube, transported at room temperature, and then stored at 20 ℃ until processing (dried saliva).

CMV serostatus of mothers was determined by CMV IgG testing on infant DBS using the SeraQuest enzyme linked immunosorbent assay (Dspoken, FL) since infant IgG reflects maternal IgG.

Congenital CMV infection was identified by the detection of CMV DNA in the collected saliva or DBS specimens. All laboratory testing was done in the central laboratory of Shandong provincial CDC with local staff trained by US CDC laboratory staff. DNA was eluted from swabs with Extracta (Beverly, MA) and extracted from DBS using thermal shock. [15] Real-time PCR was performed with TaqMan-based primers and probes targeting the viral glycoprotein B gene on Mx3000P qPCR Systems (Agilent Technologies, Santa Clara, CA). [15] For quality control, all PCR raw data were reviewed by US CDC laboratory staff, and all CMV PCR positive specimens were retested by US CDC laboratory staff with at least 100 randomly selected PCR negative specimens during annual site visits. Positive results were defined as ≥5 copies of CMV DNA per PCR reaction for saliva or ≥1 copies of CMV DNA for DBS.

2.3 Statistical analyses

The 95% confidence intervals (CIs) for the estimates of CMV seroprevalence were calculated on the assumption of a binomial distribution with normal approximation, and Poisson distribution was assumed for the prevalence of congenital CMV infection. The association of categorical or continuous factors with CMV seroprevalence and congenital CMV infection was examined using Pearson or Fisher Chi-square test, or student test, as appropriate, and by logistic regression for multivariable analysis. The real-time PCR results of the DBS and dried saliva specimens were compared with those of wet saliva specimens. Sensitivity, specificity, and predictive values for the PCR assays were calculated using standard methods for proportions and their 95% CIs were calculated with the efficient-score method. [16] All analyses were carried out with SAS V9.3 (SAS Institute, Cary, NC), and statistical significance was defined as $P < 0.05$.

China CDC Ethics Committee on Human Subjects reviewed and approved the project.

3. Results

3.1 Maternal CMV seroprevalence and prevalence of congenital CMV infection

A total of 5020 infants had DBS collected for CMV IgG testing, of which 4827 were positive for a maternal seroprevalence of 96.2% (95% CI: 95.6%—96.7%). No factors were found significantly associated with maternal CMV seroprevalence except maternal county of residence; however, the absolute difference was small and unlikely to be of practical significance (97.0% vs 95.2% for Wendeng and Pingyin Counties, respectively; $P = 0.001$).

CMV DNA was detected in the saliva or blood of 75 infants out of 10,933 infants screened for an overall prevalence of congenital CMV infection of 0.7% (95% CI: 0.5%—0.9%), with prevalences of 0.4% (14/3995), 0.6% (66/10, 857), and 0.7% (52/7761) among DBS, wet, and dried saliva specimens screened, respectively. Prevalence of congenital CMV infection decreased with increasing maternal age (0.9%, 0.6%, and 0.3% among newborns delivered from mothers aged 16—25, 26—35, and > 35 years, respectively; $P = 0.03$) (Table 1). Congenital CMV infection was not associated with county of birth ($P = 0.05$), or being born to a mother who had a previous live birth ($P = 0.36$), lived with a child aged 6 years of age ($P = 0.60$), or had occupational contact with young children ($P = 0.44$).

Congenital CMV infection was twice as prevalent among preterm infants as full term infants (1.3% vs 0.6%, $P = 0.04$). Infants with IUGR were more likely to have congenital CMV infection than those without (1.8% vs 0.7%, $P = 0.03$). Singleton pregnancies were significantly less likely to have congenital CMV infection than those pregnancies of twins or triplets (0.7% vs 2.8%, $P = 0.04$) (Table 2).

Table 1   Association of maternal factors with congenital CMV infection among 10 933 infants tested in 2 counties of Shandong Province, China, 2011 to 2013

	Congenital CMV infection		P
	Positive, n(%)	Negative, n(%)	
Overall	75(0.7)	10 858(99.3)	
Maternal age in years			0.03
16~25	39(0.9)	4 415(99.1)	
26~35	34(0.6)	5 804(99.4)	
>35	2(0.3)	639(99.7)	
Study site			0.05
Pingyin County	42(0.9)	4 878(99.1)	
Wendeng County	33(0.5)	5 980(99.5)	
Born to mother who had a previous live birth			0.36
Yes	40(0.6)	6 357(99.4)	
No	35(0.8)	4 501(99.2)	
Born to mother living with children ⩽ 6 years at home			0.60
Yes	4(0.5)	744(99.5)	
No	71(0.7)	10 111(99.3)	
Born to working mothers with occupational contact with young children			0.44
Yes	1(0.3)	301(99.7)	
No	61(0.7)	8 581(99.3)	
Type of residence			0.42
Urban	28(0.6)	4 549(99.4)	
Rural	47(0.7)	6 309(99.3)	

CMV = cytomegalovirus

Table 2　Clinical and demographic factors by congenital CMV infection status among 10 933 infants tested in 2 counties of Shandong Province, China, 2011 to 2013

	Congenital CMV infection		P
	Positive, n(%)	Negative, n(%)	
Preterm birth(≤37 weeks)			0.04
Yes	10(1.3)	783(98.7)	
No	65(0.6)	10 074(99.4)	
Sex			0.21
Male	33(0.6)	5 558(99.4)	
Female	42(0.8)	5 300(99.2)	
Intrauterine growth restriction			0.03
Yes	5(1.8)	280(98.2)	
No	70(0.7)	10 577(99.3)	
Type of delivery			0.34
Vaginal delivery	25(0.5)	4 671(99.5)	
Assisted vaginal delivery with vacuum extraction or forceps	16(1.2)	1 337(98.8)	
C-section	34(0.7)	4 849(99.3)	
Any injury during laboring			0.70
Yes	0(0.0)	21(100.0)	
No	75(0.7)	10 837(99.3)	
Perinatal asphyxia			0.61
Yes	0(0.0)	37(100.0)	
No	75(0.7)	10 821(99.3)	
Singleton pregnancy			0.04
Yes	70(0.7)	10 658(99.3)	
No	3(2.8)	106(97.2)	
Muscular force after birth			0.11
Normal	74(0.7)	10 824(99.3)	
Weak	1(2.9)	33(97.1)	
Microcephaly			0.62
Yes	0(0.0)	36(100.0)	
No	37(0.7)	5 326(99.3)	
Jaundice at birth			0.99
Yes	2(0.7)	292(99.3)	
No	73(0.7)	10 566(99.3)	
Petechiae at birth			NA
Yes	0(0.0)	0(0.0)	

(Continued)

	Congenital CMV infection		P
	Positive，n(%)	Negative，n(%)	
No	10 858(99.3)	75(0.7)	
Seizures at birth			0.87
Yes	0(0.0)	4(100.0)	
No	37(0.7)	5 358(99.3)	
Newborn hearing screening results			0.17
Normal	73(0.7)	10 123(99.3)	
Abnormal	2(0.3)	713(99.7)	
Body length at birth，cm：mean(SD)	49.7(2.9)	50.3(1.8)	0.003
Chest circumference，cm：mean(SD)	34.0(1.7)	33.62(1.9)	0.31

CMV = cytomegalovirus，SD = standard deviation

3.2　Clinical manifestations of congenital CMV infection

None of the 75 newborns with CMV infection were born with symptoms associated with congenital CMV infection. Although infants with congenital CMV infection had statistically significantly shorter body lengths than uninfected infants, the absolute difference was small (49.7 vs 50.3 cm) and unlikely to be of clinical significance. There was no difference in the prevalence of jaundice between infants with and without congenital CMV infection ($P = 0.99$) or in the occurrence of seizures ($P = 0.87$) during the newborn hospitalization. Two (2.7%) infants with congenital CMV infection failed newborn hearing screening; both failed in both ears. However, there was no difference in the proportions of infants with and without congenital CMV infection who failed newborn hearing screening ($P = 0.17$) (Table 2).

3.3　PCR results by specimen type

A total of 7 720 infants had both wet and dried saliva specimens tested, and 3 953 had both wet saliva and DBS tested. Compared with wet saliva, the sensitivity of the dried saliva was 93.9% (95% CI：82.1%—98.4%) and the specificity was 99.9% (95% CI：99.8%—100.0%). Compared with wet saliva, the sensitivity of the DBS was 39.3% (95% CI：22.1%—59.3%) and the specificity was 99.9% (95% CI：99.8%—100.0%) (Table 3). The mean CMV viral load in DBS was 2.7×10^3 copies/mL (interquartile range：$1.7 \times 10^3 - 3.9 \times 10^3$), significantly lower than the DBS viral loads from a population sample of 3 972 US newborns using identical lab method (1.0×10^4 copies/mL，$P < 0.001$). [17]

Table 3 Comparison of dried blood spots and dried saliva specimens with wet saliva specimens in screening for congenital cytomegalovirus infection in 2 counties of Shandong Province, China, 2011 to 2013

Wet saliva	Dried blood spots (N = 3 953)		Dried saliva (N = 7 720)	
	Positive	Negative	Positive	Negative
Positive	11	17	46	3
Negative	3	3 922	6	7 665
Sensitivity (95% CI)	39.3%(22.1%—59.3%)		93.9%(82.1%—94.4%)	
Specificity (95% CI)	99.9%(99.8%—100.0%)		99.9%(99.8%—100.0%)	
Positive predictive value (95% CI)	78.6%(48.8%—94.3%)		88.5%(75.9%—95.2%)	
Negative predictive value (95% CI)	99.6%(99.4%—99.8%)		100.0%(99.9%—100.0%)	

4. Discussion

Our findings of high maternal CMV seroprevalence in Shandong Province are consistent with results from studies conducted within the past 2 decades across China,[12,18-20] and suggest that high CMV seroprevalence may be ubiquitous across China. The prevalence of congenital CMV infection was 0.7% in Shandong Province, China, and no newborns with symptomatic congenital CMV infection were identified. Our findings of higher CMV prevalence among infants with low birth weight, IUGR, preterm birth, or nonsingleton pregnancy are consistent with reports from populations of other countries. [11,17,21-23]

Although the prevalence of congenital CMV infection is generally higher in populations with higher maternal seroprevalence,[9] it varies substantially across populations with high seroprevalence (0.6%—6.1%).[8] Differences in laboratory methods, and study enrollment criteria probably account for some of these reported variations.[8] More importantly, differences in socioeconomic status and exposure to young children likely affect chances of reinfection and transmission within populations with high seroprevalence. The 0.7% congenital CMV infection prevalence that we report from China is significantly lower than that reported in 2 other large studies with good ascertainment methods conducted in populations with high seroprevalence in Brazil (1.1%, n = 8047, $P = 0.003$) and Turkey (1.9%, n = 944, $P = 0.001$).[11,22] The population we examined in China had much less exposure to young children (<7% in current study) than other populations as a result of China's unique 1-child policy. This is consistent with the lower IgM seroprevalence previously reported in China (0.5%) compared to Brazil (2.3%) among females of reproductive age.[12,24] Moreover, the prevalence estimate of congenital CMV infection in the current study was similar to the recent reported prevalence (0.6%)

among 4 447 Brazilian newborns,[25] and lower than 1.1% previously reported[11] from the same investigators in the same Brazilian population. These findings echo the recent systematic review of reported variations in congenital CMV infection across developing countries.[8]

The prevalence of symptomatic congenital CMV infection might truly be lower in China than in other populations with high maternal seroprevalence. A study conducted in Beijing also failed to detect any newborns with symptomatic congenital CMV infection.[26] Although the Beijing study relied solely on DBS to identify infected infants, which has lower sensitivity compared to saliva,[27] DBS testing in that study would likely have identified infants at higher risk for symptoms and sequelae.[28]

Our finding that dried saliva is a reliable type of specimen for identifying congenital CMV infection has important public health implications in that dried saliva is much easier and more economical to store and transport than wet saliva. In populations with high maternal seroprevalence in Brazil, saliva was found to be as sensitive and specific as urine for newborn screening for congenital CMV infection and to be more easily collected than urine specimens.[29] DBS showed relatively low sensitivity of 39% compared to saliva for the detection of congenital CMV infection in China. Consistent with this finding, the mean CMV viral load in DBS from Chinese infants was 2.7×10^3, far lower than reported for DBS or blood from US infants: 1×10^4 copies/mL that used identical laboratory methods[17] and 8×10^4 copies/mL reported for asymptomatic infants (both $P < 0.001$) The relatively low CMV viral loads in CMV-infected Chinese newborns may explain the absence of symptomatic congenital CMV infection in our study. Recent study has suggested that screening with DBS may enrich for infants with the high risk of developing sequelae.[31] From a public health standpoint, screening tests for CMV that do not identify all infected infants but do identify those at higher risk for sequelae may be advantageous since 80% to 85% of infants will never develop sequelae.[31] However, it is not yet known whether DBS testing can provide adequate sensitivity for CMV screening.

Several limitations should be considered in interpreting our findings. The prevalence of congenital CMV infection was assessed with testing on multiple specimens which might increase the detecting probability and lead to overestimation. In addition, some unenrolled newborns had been transferred to other hospitals as the results of newborn diseases who were more likely to have congenital CMV infection, though the number was small and would not make much change on the estimate. In addition, the study sites were located in the relatively developed region of China and the findings might not be generalizable to the resource-limited regions where the prevalence of congenital CMV infection was reported very high,[32] and further studies are needed to verify the reported geographic variation and examine the associated risk factors. In summary, we carried out the first population-based newborn screening study for congenital CMV infection in China. In this relatively developed region of China, we found lower prevalence and milder manifestations of congenital CMV infection than seen in populations from other countries with high maternal CMV seroprevalence, suggesting that disabilities from congenital CMV infection could be relatively low in China. These findings provide additional evidence that the epidemiology of congenital CMV infection varies across populations with high maternal seroprevalence. These data also suggest that while high maternal prevalence seems to be fairly consistently associated with high prevalence of congenital CMV infection, more data on congenital CMV infection in different populations with high seroprevalence are needed for developing population-specific prevention strategies in the world.

Acknowledgments

The authors thank the help from the medical staff of the birthing hospitals in this study and the efforts of the local CDC staff in coordination, specimen storage and transportation, and performing data quality checks. The authors also thank the parents for their involvement and willingness to have their children participate in this project.

Task 5 *Scan the QR code and read the abstracts of the seven SCI papers in Appendix Ⅱ. Then check whether their writings follow the requirements stipulated by the journal.*

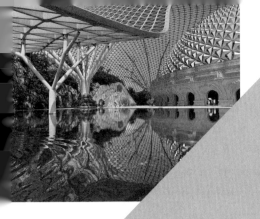

Chapter Seven

Introduction Writing

✓参考答案
✓课件申请
✓学术资源

Introduction is the first main section of the body of an academic research paper, especially SCI, which aims to provide readers with the research background and theoretical basis, and to present the questions, the hypothesis, thesis statement and the importance of the research topic. However, the writing of the introduction part often turns out to be hard and difficult in an academic paper, and there are many misunderstandings about introduction writing.

7.1　The function and importance of an introduction

As the first section of the main text, the introduction sets tone for the readers by giving essential ideas of the content and the stance of the writer. It also informs its readers how the paper is organized or how the research work is performed. The introduction in EAP provides readers with the necessary knowledge to understand the paper and its importance. It points out the main research issues and theoretical basis of the research, and clarifies the purpose of the research.

A well-written introduction of an academic paper has two general functions: one is to attract the readers' interest, encouraging the readers to continue reading the paper; the other is to provide necessary and adequate information, preparing readers for understanding the paper and evaluating the value of research. That is to say, the main function of introduction is to present readers an attractive and valuable hypothesis, while the other elements, including background, questions and importance, serve as a preparation for the readers to understand and value the hypothesis better.

Introduction shows the connections between the paper and relevant researches, and initially illustrates the significance and value of the paper. It has an important guiding significance for readers to understand the paper. At the same time, introduction defines the main issues studied in the paper and elaborates the purpose in the research, providing readers with a commanding point to grasp the pulse of the whole paper. The introduction makes it easy for the readers to understand the following parts of the text, such as materials, methods, results and discussions.

[Sample 1]

(1) The COVID-19 pandemic has made the development of a safe, effective, and deployable vaccine a critical global priority. (2) However, our understanding of immune correlates of protection to SARS-CoV-2 is currently very limited but is essential for the development of SARS-CoV-2 vaccines and other immunotherapeutic interventions. (3) To facilitate the preclinical evaluation of vaccine candidates, we recently developed a rhesus macaque model of SARS-CoV-2 infection. (4) In the present study, we constructed a set of

prototype DNA vaccines expressing various forms of the SARS-CoV-2 spike (S) protein and assessed their immunogenicity and protective efficacy against SARS-CoV-2 viral challenge in rhesus macaques. (Yu et al., 2020)

[**Analysis**]

This is a paper on SARS-CoV-2 vaccine research and development, entitled "DNA vaccine protection against SARS-CoV-2 in rhesus macaques" (DNA 疫苗对恒河猴 SARS-CoV-2 的保护作用).

The writing of this introduction is brief and clear. Only with four sentences, it summarizes all the necessary information on SARS-CoV-2 vaccine development for the readers, so that they can understand the readability of the paper accurately and quickly. The first sentence introduces the background and necessity of the research. The second sentence clarifies the unknown or research questions. In the third sentence, a key progress of the relevance of the study is made. Finally, the introduction shows the research purpose and briefly explains the research design or experimental methods.

7.2 The basic principles and components in EAP introduction writing

As the leading part of the main paper body, the writing of an introduction should normally be brief and clear. For example, *Science* requests for the introduction to the published paper is: "Text starts with a brief introduction describing the paper's significance, which should be intelligible to readers in various disciplines." It is pointed out by *Science* that the text begins with a brief and clear introduction that outlines the significance of the research and should be understandable to readers from various academic backgrounds. Obviously, according to *Science*, the basic function of the introduction is to point out the significance of the research, and at the same time, a good introduction should be "easy to understand" so that readers outside the field can understand the significance and importance of the research easily when reading the introduction of an EAP.

Accordingly, several important elements should be included and identified properly in the part of introduction. The basic components of writing an introduction are:

- introducing the necessary background information, reviewing the literature,
- putting forward the specific research hypothesis,
- clarifying the unknown or research questions or thesis statement,
- and briefly explaining the research design or experimental methods and the importance of the research topic.

This relatively fixed writing structural pattern helps readers get relevant information quickly. The structure of the introduction is somehow different from the other sections of the paper.

In addition, the following points are worthy of attention.

- The background part of the introduction shouldn't stray too far from the topic. It should focus on the specific field of the research.

- Avoid a simple list when reviewing previous research findings. Instead, organize your language in a logical order, such as in a chronological order or a relevance order from the general to specific.

- It is necessary to point out the unsolved or still existing problems in previous researches. It is a good transition to the current research. The present simple tense is generally used because this part mainly describes the research status of relevant fields.

- Especially, the highlight and the key element of this section is hypothesis, but it is typically placed at the end of this section rather than at the beginning of this section, which somewhat makes the structure of the introduction different from other sections of the paper.

- At the end of the introduction, the design and method of the research could also be briefly summarized to lay a good foundation for the body part. However, the details shouldn't be stated here. The past simple tense is usually used.

Although the introduction section of an academic paper presents a relatively fixed writing structural pattern, what kinds of essential components are included in the introduction may vary from journal to journal, from author to author. Anyway, it is recommended by ICMJE (International Committee Medical Journal Editors, 国际医学期刊编辑委员会) that the introduction should provide a context or background for the study, state the specific purpose or research objective of the study or observation, propose hypothesis to be tested or verified by the study or observation. Cite only directly pertinent references, and do not include data or conclusion from the work being reported.

[**Sample 2**]

Beginning in December, 2019, a cluster of cases of pneumonia with unknown cause was reported in Wuhan, in Hubei province of China. On Jan. 7, 2020, a novel coronavirus, severe acute respiratory syndrome coronavirus 2 (SARS-CoV-2; previously known as 2019-nCoV), was identified as the causative organism by Chinese facilities via deep sequencing analysis of patients' respiratory tract samples. SARS-CoV-2 has been shown to infect human respiratory epithelial cells through an interaction between the viral S protein and the angiotensin converting enzyme 2 receptor on human cells; thus, SARS-CoV-2 possesses a strong capability to infect humans.

Most of the initial cases of coronavirus disease 2019 (COVID-19), caused by SARS-CoV-2, were epidemiologically linked to exposure to Wuhan's Huanan Seafood Market, where wild animals are traded. Although the market has been closed since Jan. 1, 2020, as part of efforts to contain the outbreak, patients without exposure to the market but with a history of travel to Wuhan or close physical contact with a patient confirmed to have COVID-19, including health-care workers, have also been identified, suggesting strong human-to-human transmission. The number of cases has been increasing rapidly: by Feb. 15, 2020, more than 60 000 cases of COVID-19 pneumonia had been reported in China and in other countries worldwide (including Thailand, Japan, South Korea, and the USA), and 1 524 patients had died, equivalent to a mortality rate of around 2%.

The clinical features of the initial 41 patients confirmed to be infected with SARS-CoV-2 included lower respiratory tract illness with fever, dry cough, and dyspnoea, a manifestation similar to those of two other diseases caused by coronaviruses, severe acute respiratory syndrome (SARS) and Middle East respiratory syndrome (MERS). However, the radiological changes in the lungs of people with COVID-19 pneumonia have not been fully characterised. CT is important in the diagnosis and treatment of lung diseases. In our experience, the imaging features of COVID-19 pneumonia are diverse, ranging from normal appearance to diffuse changes in the lungs. In addition, different radiological patterns are observed at different times throughout the disease course. Because the time between onset of symptoms and the development of acute respiratory distress syndrome (ARDS) was as short as 9 days among the initial patients with COVID-19 pneumonia, early recognition of the disease is essential for the management of these patients.

We aimed to analyse the evolution of chest CT imaging features in patients with COVID-19 pneumonia, and to compare the imaging findings across the disease course, to facilitate early diagnosis of this newly emerging, life threatening infection. (Shi et al., 2020)

[**Analysis**]

This article is a clinical descriptive study on COVID-19 pneumonia in Wuhan, published on *Lancet Infect Dis* in April 2020. As we can see, the introduction to the article is written according to the recommendation of the ICMJE. The first three paragraphs provide a context or background for the study, and then, in the fourth or last paragraph, the study purposes are presented and hypothesis is proposed. The conclusion is not included in the part of the introduction.

7.3   Organization and structural discourse of an introduction

Commonly, there are mainly three types of academic researches: hypothesis-testing research, descriptive research and method research, and their introductions usually follow a relatively standard pattern of organization. It is necessary for us to understand and learn a general and standard structural pattern of the introduction section.

In terms of the structure, a well-organized introduction presents a funnel shape, called the "funnel-shaped" introduction. It begins with a broad, general statement of the research scope, and then step by step, narrow down to the research focus, such as the problems to be solved or the purpose of research.

From the viewpoint of socially communicative function of the introduction of an academic paper, and based on the linguistic research on the introduction of academic papers, Swales and Feak (2012) proposed a famous discourse pattern: the Create-a-Research-Space (or CARS) model(建立学术研究空间模型).

7.3.1 Funnel-shaped introduction

The funnel-shaped introduction moves from general information to specific information, that is to say, it begins with general research topic and then narrows down to the research topic. The general information eases the readers into the research statement by first introducing the topic. From the views of content and organization, the funnel presents a minimum of three steps: known, unknown and question. It tells the readers its story like this:

- Here's what we have known now;
- Here's what is not yet known;
- Here's the question that exists.

1) **Known**: What is to know about the topic. It is the first step to start the story line in the funnel, which starts with brief explanation of the background, and then be narrowed by appropriate scientific logic to the unknown. It is not necessary to include everything about your research scope because the specific function of the introduction is to provide only the information necessary for understanding what leads to hypothesis, and understanding the hypothesis.

2) **Unknown**: What is not known. The unknown should be just one, but it is a crucial sentence because it functions as a transition from the background to the hypothesis.

3) **Question**: It is the end of the funnel, the focal point and the hypothesis of the introduction. The background (known and unknown) is what leads to the question, and the question exactly presents the readers what will be revealed in the study.

4) **The other two additional steps**: Experimental approach and importance. The introduction can end up with the statement of the question or hypothesis or can

go on to state the experimental approach which follows from the questions, like "here is how we went about answering the question." And there are no special requirements to indicate the importance of the research. Sometimes the importance is not indicated.

[Sample 3]

（1）Laboratory mice are a mainstay of biomedical research and have been instrumental for many important discoveries in the field of immunology. （2）However, there are also major limitations, including conflicting results rooted in divergent microbiota among research facilities and the limited ability to predict the complex immune responses of humans. （3）Recent studies have shown that conventional laboratory mice are too far removed from natural environmental conditions to faithfully mirror the physiology of free-living mammals such as humans. （4）Mammals and their immune systems evolved to survive and thrive in a microbial world and behave differently in a sanitized environment. （5）To generate a mouse model that more closely resembles the natural mammalian metaorganism with coevolved microbes and pathogens, we transferred C57BL/6 embryos into wild mice. This resulted in a colony of C57BL/6 mice, which we call "wildlings." (Rosshart et al., 2019)

[Analysis]

The information in Sample 3 is organized in a "funnel". The first, third and fourth sentences are for the known information, and the second sentence is for the unknown. Then, the background (known and unknown) leads immediately to the hypothesis (the fifth sentence) followed by the experimental approach and result. Its funnel-shaped organization of the introduction section could be illustrated as follows:

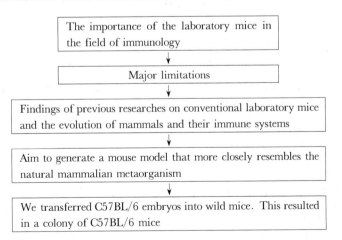

A longer introduction could also follow this shape usually by expanding the known.

7.3.2 The CARS model

Swales (1990) put forward the communicative thought that the social purpose of the introduction of academic papers is to "Create-a-Research-Space". On the basis of substantive studies of articles involving many disciplines, Swales and Feak (2012) proposed the Create-a-Research-Space model for introduction in an academic paper. It describes the rhetorical structure of the introduction of academic papers through the analysis method of "Moves and Steps"(语步及步骤). This model is a linguistic structure analysis model based on moves and steps. The CARS model provides a three-step moves for the discourse of an introduction:

Moves	Steps of the Move
Move 1: Establish a research territory	• Showing the general research area related to your study or discussion involved; • Introducing and reviewing items of previous research in the area.
Move 2: Establish a niche	• By pointing out the problems, questions, limitations and contradictions of the previous research; • By extending or exploiting previous knowledge in some way.
Move 3: Occupy the niche	• Proposing research questions and hypotheses; • Outlining the research purposes or stating the nature of your research; • Announcing your new key findings; • Stating the significance or value of your research; • Indicating the structure of the research paper (probable in some fields, but rare in others).

In Move 1, the literature review provides the readers with the indispensable research background of relevant research fields and shows the readers like this: "Here's what we have known and what we have done."

Move 2 is to establish a niche in introduction by giving reasons for the present research. It tells the readers like: "Here's something wrong. Here's something missing and something unclear in previous work. Here's something to add." Establishing a niche is usually indicated by using transitional words or signal words like "however, challenge, there is no …, this question remains …, … still need to be …", etc. Move 2 should be established clearly and briefly. Usually, one or two sentences are enough. There're four different methods to establish a niche:

- counter-claiming (indicating negative evaluation or showing weakness in previous researches);
- indicating a gap in previous research (something missing);
- raising a question about previous research (something unclear or ambiguous);
- continuing a tradition (extending previous research).

In Move 3, research hypotheses and purposes are proposed directly or indirectly. It tells the readers like: "Here's the thing we want to do, here's the way we supposed to deal with that questions and here's the key."

[**Sample 4**]

(1) Heart failure (HF) is a significant health issue affecting approximately 5.7 million adults in the United States with estimated annual costs of over \$30 billion. (2) About one quarter of the patients discharged with a primary diagnosis of HF are readmitted within 30 days. (3) Hospital readmissions are associated with significant additional cost and adverse clinical outcomes. (4) The Center for Medicare and Medicaid Services (CMS) Hospital Readmissions Reduction Program provides financial incentives to hospitals to reduce readmissions for these patients. (5) As a result, significant attention and effort has been put into reducing readmission of HF patients. (6) Identifying HF patients at high risk for hospital readmission is crucial for targeting interventions to reduce readmissions. (7) Several prior studies predicted 30-day readmission, although the predictive accuracy of these models is limited. (8) Since the outcome of interest is 30-day readmission for any cause, it is possible that non-cardiovascular risk factors play an important role. (9) While prior studies looked at socioeconomic and psychosocial characteristics, there is limited information on non-cardiovascular risk factors predicting 30-day readmission. (10) Therefore, in the present study, we aimed to develop a predictive model for HF readmissions including parameters reflecting non-cardiovascular disease (CVD) burden, using a novel statistical bootstrap LASSO approach for variable selection. (11) In addition, we examined the specific reasons, including non-cardiovascular diagnoses, for which HF patients are readmitted within 30 days following HF hospitalization discharge. (Kutyifa et al., 2018)

[**Analysis**]

1. Establish the research territory

1) Research field related to the study: sentences 1 – 2.

2) Reviewing previous work or effort done in this regard: sentences 3 – 4.

3) The consequence: sentence 5.

2. Establish the niche

1) Pointing out the problem needed to be solved: sentence 6.

2) Extending or exploiting previous knowledge: sentences 7 – 9.

    Achievements: "Several prior studies predicated 30-day readmission";

        "non-cardiovascular risk factors play an important role";

        "the prior studies looked at socioeconomic and psychosocial characteristics".

    Limitations: "The predictive accuracy of these models is limited";

        "there is limited information on non-cardiovascular risk factors predicting 30-day readmission."

3. Occupy the niche (sentences 10 – 11)

1) Proposing research purpose/hypotheses/new key findings: sentence 10.

2) Significance or value of the research: sentence 11.

Chapter Review

In this chapter we have discussed how to understand and write the introduction section that conforms to international norms, involving the functions, the basic principles and components, and the organization and structural discourse.

1. The basic components of an introduction are:
   - Introducing the necessary background information, reviewing the literature;
   - Putting forward the specific research hypothesis;
   - Clarifying the unknown or research questions or thesis statements;
   - Briefly explaining the research design or experimental methods and the importance of the research topic.

2. In terms of structure, a well-organized introduction presents a funnel shape, beginning with a broad, general statement of the research scope, and then narrowing down to the research focus.

3. In order to write an effective introduction, Swales and Feak (2012) identified a three-move pattern in the introduction section of most papers, and proposed a famous discourse pattern called the Creating-a-Research-Space (or CARS) model which contains three moves:

   Move 1: Establishing a research territory;

   Move 2: Establishing a niche;

   Move 3: Occupying the niche.

Assignments

Task 1   *The following sentences are taken from the introduction section of an academic paper entitled "General ecological models for human subsistence, health and poverty", published in* **Nature**. *Rearrange these sentences into a coherent introduction by numbering them from 1 to 10.*

_____ A. We use this general modelling structure as a blueprint to derive a library of models of increasing complexity to represent specific ecological, economic and epidemiological systems that investigators can apply to systems of interest.

_____ B. The conclusion of the Millennium Development era in 2015 provided benchmarks for human development, including a target to reduce extreme poverty by 50%. As nearly a billion people in the world still subsist below the international poverty line, there remains considerable debate over general causes of persistent extreme poverty.

_____ C. Using simple toy models based on such principles, a recent study demonstrated that under specific assumptions, ecologically driven poverty traps can be formed. These models were not analysed broadly to provide a general understanding of how such models behave and did not reveal general conditions that lead to poverty traps.

_____ D. As the global health community has broadened its priorities in light of the sustainable development goals and a movement for planetary health, these statistics underline the importance of understanding ecological foundations of economic development based on two core principles: (1) the capital of the poor is often biological in the form of crops, livestock, forests, wildlife, soils and fisheries; and (2) the dynamics of capital is embedded within systems of ecological interactions or food webs that include pathogens of humans and their biological resources.

_____ E. Approximately 70% of the poor in sub-Saharan Africa and Southeast Asia subsist from primary resource extraction: agriculture, timber and fishing. Concomitant to this, around 35% suffer from chronic malnutrition and more than 75% die from infectious diseases.

_____ F. Here, we present the first general theoretical framework of its kind where ecological, economic and epidemiological factors leading to persistent poverty are generalized and broadly analysed. We show that systems of capital (renewable resources, human capital, physical capital) and natural enemies (for example, infectious diseases and pests) can be described with two fundamental equations, comparable to predator-prey models in population biology.

_____ G. "Poverty traps" commonly refer to the idea that accumulating wealth requires a minimum amount of wealth (for example, beyond subsistence), such that there is enough to be saved and invested for the future. Modern (neoclassical) economic growth theory has shown how poverty traps can arise from nonlinear processes in the growth rate of capital (or wealth).

_____ H. Most models of poverty traps are phenomenological—that is, based on qualitative assumptions about these nonlinear processes—and are rarely derived from explicit understanding of the underlying feedbacks that reinforce poverty, such as disease and resource scarcity. Owing to effects on child development and labour productivity, the role of health conditions (particularly disease and malnutrition) as a driver of poverty traps has gained increasing attention.

_____ I. These models are then parameterized from country-level data and analysed over the feasible parameter space to explore qualitative and quantitative properties of different regimes of economic development and human health. The analyses show that poverty traps, defined as self-reinforcing (that is, stable equilibrium) systems of poverty, are general features of the models.

_____ J. It has also been recognized that poverty is an important risk factor for acquiring and succumbing to disease. The intuitive argument for these coupled disease-poverty systems is that escaping from such traps is difficult for the rural poor, who are highly susceptible to infectious diseases and rely heavily on subsistence agriculture. Notably, human health and resource dynamics are determined by biological processes that are well studied in the scientific literature. Models of the ecological basis of human livelihoods can accordingly be coupled explicitly with economics to identify dynamics that are based on fewer, simpler and more evidence-based assumptions that are rooted in scientific knowledge.

Task 2 *Read the following titles of some SCI papers and their opening sentences in their introductions, then match each opening sentence with its appropriate title by writing the number on the left side of the title.*

Titles	Opening sentences
A. Environment Changes Genetic Effects on Respiratory Conditions and Allergic Phenotypes	1. Social and political tensions keep on fueling armed conflicts around the world. Although each conflict is the result of an individual context-specific mixture of interconnected factors, ethnicity appears to play a prominent and almost ubiquitous role in many of them.
B. Study of Epidemiological Aspects of Hyperuricemia in Poland	2. An estimated 250 million people worldwide are chronically infected with hepatitis B virus (HBV), which is often asymptomatic during the early stages of disease.
C. Future Urban Land Expansion and Implications for Global Croplands	3. The results of recent epidemiological studies show that hyperuricemia affects millions of people.

(Continued)

Titles	Opening sentences
D. Armed-conflict Risks Enhanced by Climate-related Disasters in Ethnically Fractionalized Countries	4. The global prevalence of asthma and other allergic conditions such as rhinitis, dermatitis and atopy, have been increasing for the past 30 to 40 years
E. Cost-effectiveness of Community-Based Screening and Treatment for Chronic Hepatitis B in the Gambia: An Economic Modelling Analysis	5. Urban expansion often occurs on croplands. However, there is little scientific understanding of how global patterns of future urban expansion will affect the world's cultivated areas.

Task 3 *According to the CARS model（Swales & Feak, 2012）, there're four different methods to establish a niche: counter-claiming, indicating a gap in previous research, raising a question about previous research and continuing a tradition. Below, there are three introductions, selected from SCI papers. Please read introductions 1, 2 and 3 and pick out the niche-sentence or niche-sentences from each introduction, and then tell which kind of method they belong to.*

[Introduction 1]

Infectious diseases such as pneumonia and diarrhoea are major contributors to child morbidity and mortality in low- and middle-income countries, with most cases occurring in the first 2 years of life. These diseases are associated with a high economic burden. In Southeast Asia, after excluding neonatal deaths, pneumonia and diarrhoea account for half of all deaths in children under 5 years of age.

Environmental tobacco smoke（ETS）exposure is an important and early modifiable risk factor for childhood illnesses such as respiratory symptoms, respiratory infections, asthma and sudden infant death. The biological mechanisms of the disease risk conferred by ETS exposure have been investigated by in vitro functional studies on Toll-like receptors and blood cells, and these studies have suggested that tobacco smoke alters local and systemic innate immunity. Therefore, the effect of ETS exposure may not be limited to respiratory diseases. However, there is limited and conflicting evidence regarding the association of ETS exposure with the risks of other types of infectious diseases such as acute otitis media and gastroenteritis. Furthermore, few prospective studies of child populations have assessed the risks associated with ETS exposure in populations in which the contribution of female or maternal smoking exposure is negligible like Vietnamese. We previously reported that ETS exposure due to household members was significantly associated with an increased risk of parent-reported child pneumonia (OR = 1. 55, 95% CI: 1.25—1.92) in a cross-sectional population surveillance study in Vietnam; however, the detection of cases was not fully reliable because it was based on parental self-report questionnaires. As tobacco smoking is highly prevalent among young Vietnamese men and as only 1. 0% of smokers in Nha Trang, Vietnam, are women 18—50 years of age, parental smoking, particularly paternal smoking, could be a risk factor for childhood diseases including, but not limited to, respiratory infections.

In the present study, we described the burden and pattern of severe illness including infectious and non-infectious diseases that require hospitalization using the medical records of Vietnamese children registered in a prospective birth cohort study. Additionally, we aimed to improve the strength of evidence for the association of parental smoking with the incidence of childhood health problems. (Miyahara et al. 2018)

[Introduction 2]

Atrial fibrillation (AF) is the most common cardiac arrhythmia. The treatment approach for AF includes either restoration and maintenance of sinus rhythm or ensuring adequate ventricular rate control. Maintainance of sinus rhythm may be provided by anti-arrhythmic drugs (AADs) or catheter ablation. Catheter ablation of AF is recommended for patients with symptomatic paroxysmal atrial fibrillation (PAF) despite AADs[1]. Pulmonary vein isolation (PVI) has become a major curative measure of AF in drug resistant patients[2, 3]. Radiofrequency (RF) ablation is widely accepted as an effective treatment for PAF. Performing point-by-point ablation using RF energy is challenging. Cryoenergy by cryoballoon technique is an alternative to RF ablation. Balloon-based cryoenergy for PVI simplifies the reliable creation of a complete circumferential lesion around the pulmonary veins (PV) with only a limited number of applications. Cryoballoon ablation is safe, and has a similar success rate, when compared to RF ablation with comparable procedure and fluoroscopy times in patients suffering from PAF[4]. However, reported 1 year success rates are limited to 60%—74%[5-8]. Therefore, the aim of this study is to identify the predictors of success specifically in patients undergoing cryoballoon ablation for PAF. (Evranos et al. , 2013)

[Introduction 3]

HIV/AIDS is a leading cause of morbidity and mortality in sub-Saharan Africa. In the nearly four decades since HIV was first recognized, scientific breakthroughs have transformed the once invariably fatal illness to one that can be successfully managed with lifelong anti-retroviral therapy (ART). Despite the rapid increase in the use of ART since the mid-2000s and the resulting decline in mortality, 34% of people in east and southern Africa and 60% of people in west and central Africa who are living with HIV are not currently receiving any treatment and HIV/AIDS remains the most common cause of death in sub-Saharan Africa. The burden of the global HIV epidemic is disproportionately concentrated in sub-Saharan Africa, where—in 2017—75% of deaths and 65% of new infections occurred and where 71% of people living with HIV resided.

The global community has repeatedly called for the end of the HIV epidemic. Millennium Development Goal 6 (Combat HIV/AIDS, malaria, and other diseases) included the target: "To halt by 2015 and have started to reverse the spread of HIV/AIDS." More recently, Sustainable Development Goal 3 (Ensure healthy lives and promote well-being for all at all ages) explicitly calls for the end of the epidemic by 2030. The Joint United Nations Programme on HIV/AIDS (UNAIDS) fast-track strategy has set diagnosis and treatment targets for 2020 and 2030, with the goal of markedly reducing both new infections and deaths by 2030. Despite these goals, a recent review of the state of HIV concluded that the world is not on track to end the HIV epidemic. Moreover, global spending on HIV in sub-Saharan Africa peaked in 2013 and has since declined, potentially compromising existing efforts to combat HIV.

Renewed commitment and new tools are required to get the world on track to bring HIV infection under control, in sub-Saharan Africa and globally. Local data on the current prevalence of HIV are such a tool, providing a means to target resources and interventions more efficiently. (Dwyer-Lindgren et al., 2019)

Task 4 *Do you know how to clearly identify the subject area of interest in an introduction? Underline the key words in the title and first two sentences of the introduction of papers 2 and 3 in Appendix Ⅱ, and see how the research is highly focused.*

Task 5 *Complete the following sentences by translating the expression in parentheses into English .*

1. _____（大量的医学研究表明）that parasite infestation is a cause or contributing factor to many of the diseases plaguing mankind today.

2. The second argument is that the conventional doctrine leads to decisions concerning life and death _____（其根据是不相干的）.

3. Furthermore, _____（临床试验和动物实验研究结果表明）that these complications might progress despite glycemic control, a phenomenon termed metabolic memory.

4. _____（本研究的目的是）to determine the relationship between cervical spine immobilization and neurologic sequelae in penetrating cervical trauma.

5. This part lays a sound theoretical foundation for this research and meanwhile _____（提出了本研究的目标和假设）.

6. _____（对⋯⋯十分必要/⋯⋯具有重要意义）to create a reliable and human-like animal model of urinary tract infection (UTI) for studies of the etiology, mechanism and treatment of UTI.

7. Several groups of researchers have used disease-prone cells created in this way to _____（探索疾病的发展）, and whether it succumbs to drugs.

8. This paper introduced the recommended immunization schedule for persons aged 0—18 years old in the United States in 2008 which can _____（为旅行者预防接种提供参考和借鉴）.

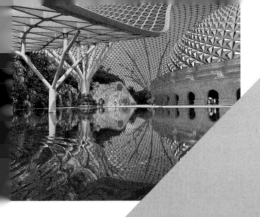

Chapter Eight

Materials and Methods Writing

Lead-in Questions

1. What information is conveyed in the section of materials and methods?

2. Can you omit the summary of materials and methods in the abstract section?

3. Do you think it is crucial to clearly explain how you carried out your study step by step? Why or why not?

4. How can the collected data be reported in this section?

5. Is it necessary to explain this section under several subheadings?

Learning Objectives

After learning this unit, you will be able to:

1. understand the principles to follow in writing materials and methods,

2. and get to know how to organize this section.

✓参考答案
✓课件申请
✓学术资源

The section of materials and methods comes after the introduction in an experimental research paper. It is the second section of the main body of the paper. Simply speaking, the materials must appropriately present what the study illustrates or clarifies and the methods should clarify what was done, how, and why.

8.1 The function of the materials and methods section

The aim of this section is to illustrate the technical path to solve the research problem. On the one hand, this section provides reference for other researchers; on the other hand, it provides basis for the reliability and credibility of research results.

For scientific research papers, the main purpose of the materials and methods section is to give full details of the methodology employed in the study and defend the reason for a particular method you have chosen over competing methods. This section translates the research question into a detailed recipe of operations. It is the foundation of a research paper and scientists are advised to begin their writing with materials and methods (Katz, 2006)

The materials and methods section mainly describes and explains the materials employed and the procedural steps used in the research in detail. In this section, it is crucial to provide enough quantitative details (what, where, how much, how long, etc.) about your protocol by which the validity of a study is ultimately judged. More importantly, by reading this section a trained researcher should be able to duplicate or reproduce your experiments and educated readers should have enough information to evaluate the efficacy of your experiments. Therefore, the author must provide a clear and precise description.

8.2 Principles and key points of the materials and methods writing

In order to get a general understanding of materials and methods writing, let's start with the basic and common writing principles that we should follow.

The general and important principle of writing materials and methods is: clear, precise and consistent. Some basic details are as follows:

- The research design or scheme should be introduced and summarized briefly and correctly.
- Tables or figures are useful devices for clarifying and summarizing the research procedure(s) or the methods for the readers.

- Experimental results shouldn't be included in this section.
- The past simple tense is usually used.
- Use subheadings to your advantage. The use of the second and third level headings gives more hierarchy to the experimental materials and methods described in this section.
- Use topic sentences to write the main points of each paragraph.
- The content of each section should be organized in a logical order, especially in chronological or importance order.
- If the research involves animals or humans, the paper must state whether the research plan has been approved by the relevant committee, or the informed consent should be attached as required by the journal.
- It is necessary to reaffirm the research question to reinforce the unity and consistence of the introduction.

The criterion for a well-written materials and methods section is that a reasonably knowledgeable colleague could repeat your experiment after reading the description. This is because the cornerstone of the scientific method requires your results to be reproducible. For the results to be judged reproducible, you must provide the basis for repetition of the experiments for others.

The following sample is a clinical descriptive study on COVID-19 pneumonia in Wuhan, published on *Lancet Infect Dis* in April 2020. Read this passage according to the above principles. Try to build an overall understanding of materials and methods writing.

[**Sample 1**]

Study design and participants

This was a retrospective study done at two centres in Wuhan. Patients with confirmed COVID-19 pneumonia who were admitted to Wuhan Jinyintan Hospital or Union Hospital of Tongji Medical College, and who underwent serial chest CT scans, were retrospectively enrolled.

In the patients who presented to Wuhan Jinyintan Hospital, SARS-CoV-2 infection was confirmed by next-generation sequencing or real-time RT-PCR, in accordance with a previously published protocol. The following primers and probe targeted to the envelope gene of SARS-CoV-2 were used: forward primer 5′-TCAGAATGCCAATCTCCCCAAC-3′; reverse primer 5′-AAAGGTCCACCCGATACATTGA-3′; probe5′-CY5CTAGTTACACTAG CCATCCTTACTGC-3′BHQ1.

The diagnosis of the cases from Union Hospital was initially based on the criteria published by WHO on Jan. 12, 2020,[12] and all cases were later confirmed by real-time RT-PCR analysis of throat swab specimens, using the same protocol as above when PCR kits were available. Based on the time interval between onset of symptoms and the CT scan, we designated four groups of patients in our study: group 1 (subclinical cases, in which CT scans were done before onset of symptoms); group 2 (CT scans done ≤ 1 week after symptom onset); group 3 (CT scans done>1 to 2 weeks after symptom onset); and group 4 (CT scans done>2 weeks to 3 weeks after symptom onset). Three readers (XH, NJ, and YF) recorded the clinical characteristics, laboratory findings, and comorbidities of the patients at the time of imaging. This study was approved by the institutional review boards of the relevant centres. The requirement for informed patient consent was waived by the ethics committee for this retrospective study.

CT image acquisition

All CT scans were obtained with patients in the supine position, using one of the following scanners: SOMATOM Perspective, SOMATOM Spirit, or SOMATOM Definition AS + (Siemens Healthineers, Forchheim, Germany). Scans were done from the level of the upper thoracic inlet to the inferior level of the costophrenic angle, and the following parameters were used: detector collimation widths 64 mm×0.6 mm, 128 mm×0.6 mm, 64 mm×0.6 mm, and 64 mm×0.6 mm; and tube voltage 120 kV. The tube current was regulated by an automatic exposure control system (CARE Dose 4D; Siemens Healthineers). Images were reconstructed with a slice thickness of 1.5 mm or 1 mm and an interval of 1.5 mm or 1 mm, respectively. The reconstructed images were transmitted to the workstation and picture archiving and communication systems (PACS) for multiplanar reconstruction post-processing.

Table 1 Clinical characteristics and laboratory findings of patients with COVID-19 pneumonia

	All patients (n = 81)	Group 1 (n = 15)	Group 2 (n = 21)	Group 3 (n = 30)	Group 4 (n = 15)	P value*
Characteristics						
Age, years	49.5(11.0)	44.9(9.0)	48.8(13.0)	52.3(13.0)	49.5(11.0)	0.277 8
>50	40(49%)	4(27%)	10(48%)	19(63%)	7(47%)	0.144 4
≤50	41(51%)	11(73%)	11(52%)	11(37%)	8(53%)	...
Sex	...	...	...	...	...	0.087 1
Male	42(52%)	4(27%)	11(52%)	20(67%)	7(47%)	...
Female	39(48%)	11(73%)	10(48%)	10(33%)	8(53%)	...
History of exposure to Huanan Market	31(38%)	0	8(38%)	14(47%)	9(60%)	0.001 3
Symptoms						
Fever	59(73%)	0	18(86%)	27(90%)	14(93%)	<0.000 1
Maximum temperature, ℃	...	36.6(0.1)	38.1(0.8)	38.2(0.8)	38.5(0.7)	<0.000 1

(**Continued**)

	All patients (n = 81)	Group 1 (n = 15)	Group 2 (n = 21)	Group 3 (n = 30)	Group 4 (n = 15)	P value*
≤37.3	24(30%)	15(100%)	3(14%)	5(17%)	1(7%)	<0.000 1
37.3—38	20(25%)	0	9(43%)	8(27%)	3(20%)	⋯
38—39	23(28%)	0	7(33%)	11(37%)	5(33%)	⋯
>39	14(17%)	0	2(10%)	6(20%)	6(40%)	⋯
Dyspnoea	34(42%)	0	9(43%)	13(43%)	12(80%)	<0.000 1
Chest tightness	18(22%)	0	5(24%)	7(23%)	6(40%)	0.046 7
Cough	48(59%)	0	15(71%)	21(70%)	12(80%)	<0.000 1
Sputum	15(19%)	0	3(14%)	6(20%)	6(40%)	0.038 5
Rhinorrhea	21(26%)	0	5(24%)	10(33%)	6(40%)	0.027 9
Anorexia	1(1%)	0	1(5%)	0	0	0.629 6
Weakness	7(9%)	0	1(5%)	4(13%)	2(13%)	0.406 5
Vomiting	4(5%)	0	2(10%)	2(7%)	0	0.577 7
Headache	5(6%)	0	2(10%)	2(7%)	1(7%)	0.864 5
Dizziness	2(2%)	0	0	1(3%)	1(7%)	0.805 6
Diarrhoea	3(4%)	0	1(5%)	1(3%)	1(7%)	1.000 0
Laboratory results						
Leukocyte count, $\times 10^9$/L	8.1(3.4)	8.0(2.5)	7.8(3.6)	8.4(3.5)	8.2(4.2)	0.933 7
<10	55(68%)	12(80%)	14(67%)	19(63%)	10(67%)	0.764 7
≥10	26(32%)	3(20%)	7(33%)	11(37%)	5(33%)	⋯
Lymphocyte count, $\times 10^9$/L	1.1(0.3)	1.1(0.3)	1.0(0.3)	1.1(0.3)	1.1(0.3)	0.855 7
<1.0	27(33%)	3(20%)	9(43%)	11(37%)	4(27%)	0.494 1
≥1.0	54(67%)	12(80%)	12(57%)	19(63%)	11(73%)	⋯
Platelet count, $\times 10^9$/L	212.2 (99.7)	202.9 (67.4)	213.5 (100.8)	206.8 (96.1)	230.5 (134.8)	0.872 3
<100	0	0	0	0	0	⋯
≥100	81(100%)	15(100%)	21(100%)	30(100%)	15(100%)	⋯
Haemoglobin, ng/mL	123.9 (12.0)	125.1 (13.5)	126.7 (13.4)	119.6 (12.8)	124.8 (9.1)	0.649 4
C-reactive protein, mg/L	47.6(41.8)	6.9(5.4)	61.4(39.6)	71.3(39.8)	49.8(42.4)	0.005 1
Serum amyloid A protein, mg/L	213.5 (177.8)	143.3 (108.4)	257.6 (264.2)	216.6 (66.7)	NA	0.330 0

(Continued)

	All patients (n=81)	Group 1 (n=15)	Group 2 (n=21)	Group 3 (n=30)	Group 4 (n=15)	P value*
Alanine aminotransferase, U/L	46.2(29.5)	30.8(8.9)	50.6(24.8)	48.7(33.1)	50.6(37.7)	0.162 9
Aspartate aminotransferase, U/L	40.8(17.9)	30.2(8.7)	47.7(20.8)	42.7(18.0)	37.8(16.4)	0.002 6
≤40	38(47%)	11(73%)	8(38%)	12(40%)	7(47%)	0.158 6
>40	43(53%)	4(27%)	13(62%)	18(60%)	8(53%)	...
Total bilirubin, μmol/L	11.9(3.6)	9.2(0.6)	14.1(4.3)	11.9(3.9)	NA	0.452 6
Albumin, g/L	32.9(8.1)	NA	34.0(9.3)	30.1(2.8)	NA	0.566 6
Glucose, mmol/L	6.4(2.1)	6.4(5.0)	5.2(1.9)	6.8(1.6)	NA	0.871 3
Creatinine, μmol/L	75.4(29.8)	63.7(16.5)	68.0(15.4)	115.4(46.2)	58.4(1.3)	0.180 3
Prothrombin time, s	10.7(0.9)	10.6(0.9)	10.5(0.4)	10.7(1.0)	10.9(1.6)	0.902 2
Activated partial thromboplastin time, s	32.1(7.6)	26.9(3.9)	34.3(6.7)	34.5(13.1)	29.2(2.4)	0.481 4
Thrombin time, s	28.9(8.4)	21.8(5.4)	32.3(8.2)	24.9(7.6)	32.3(7.9)	0.316 9
Fibrinogen, g/L	1.5(2.3)	0.7(0.3)	1.92(3.5)	2.3(3.0)	0.3(0.1)	0.796 0
D-dimers, mg/L	6.5(0.8)	6.5(0.3)	6.9(1.1)	5.8(0.2)	NA	0.494 0
Comorbidities						
Any	21(26%)	4(27%)	5(24%)	9(30%)	3(20%)	0.939 7
Chronic pulmonary disease	9(11%)	1(7%)	3(14%)	3(10%)	2(13%)	0.894 5
Diabetes	10(12%)	3(20%)	2(10%)	3(10%)	2(13%)	0.800 5
Hypertension	12(15%)	2(13%)	1(5%)	7(23%)	2(13%)	0.357 1
Chronic renal failure	3(4%)	0	0	3(10%)	0	0.310 1
Cardiovascular disease	8(10%)	3(20%)	1(5%)	3(10%)	1(7%)	0.549 4
Cerebrovascular disease	6(7%)	1(7%)	1(5%)	3(10%)	1(7%)	0.936 7
Malignancy	4(5%)	1(7%)	1(5%)	2(7%)	0	0.914 8
Hepatitis or liver cirrhosis	7(9%)	0	2(10%)	3(10%)	2(13%)	0.681 2

Data are mean(SD) or n(%). NA = not available. * Difference among groups 1~4.

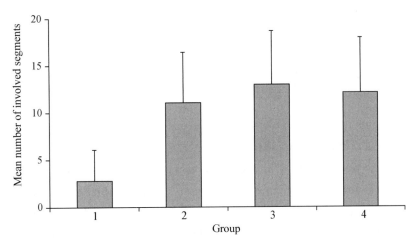

Figure 1：Number of involved lung segments at various timepoints from symptom onset
Bars show the mean number of involved lung segments on CT scans from patients in group 1 (scan before symptom onset; n = 15), group 2 (scan ≤1 week after symptom onset; n = 21), group 3 (scan >1 week to 2 weeks after symptom onset; n = 30), and group 4 (scan >2 weeks to 3 weeks after symptom onset; n = 15).

Image interpretation

Images from cases seen at Union Hospital were analysed by two radiologists (HS ［a senior thoracic radiologist with 30 years' experience］ and XH ［a radiology resident with 4 years' experience in interpreting chest CT images］). Images from cases seen at Wuhan Jinyintan Hospital were interpreted by two radiologists experienced in thoracic radiology (YF ［12 years' experience］ and NJ ［10 years' experience］). All Digital Imaging and Communications in Medicine (DICOM) images from the CT studies were analysed without access to clinical or laboratory findings. The evaluators independently and freely assessed the CT features using both axial CT images and multiplanar reconstruction images. After separate evaluations, any disagreements were resolved by discussion and consensus. CT imaging features recorded from our cohort are summarised in the Appendix 2(略).

Follow-up chest CT

Follow-up chest CT scans were reviewed by two radiologists (HS and YF). The images were assessed and the evolution of lesions rated as either no significant change, resolution, or progression, compared with the previous chest CT from the same patient (Appendix 2). Decisions were reached by consensus.

Statistical analysis

Analyses were done with SAS software version 9.4. Distribution normality was assessed using the Kolmogorov-Smirnov test. Normally distributed data were presented as mean (SD), non-normally distributed data as median (IQR), and categorical variables as frequency (%). CIs of proportions were calculated using the Clopper-Pearson method.

Differences between groups were analyzed by Fisher's exact test (for categorical data) or one-way ANOVA (for continuous data).

Role of the funding source

There was no funding source for this study. (Shi et al. , 2020)

[**Analysis**]

Firstly, in this section, the verb tenses are mainly in the past tense, which indicates that this section is about the completed work.

Then, this section is divided into six subheadings (Study design and participants, CT image acquisition, Image interpretation, Follow-up chest CT, Statistical analysis and Role of the funding source), giving more hierarchy to the experimental materials and methods described in this section. On the other hand, the sequence of experiments is consistent with the actual research experiments, and the related experiments are described clearly, accurately and objectively. Thus, the author's research intention is reflected clearly and effectively.

Each of the main experimental steps contains a detailed description of important experiments, providing readers in this field with important experimental parameters and an important basis for evaluating the repeatability of this study. References are also listed to make the readers well informed.

Obviously, this section is written clearly, precisely and consistently.

8.3 The organization and discourse of the materials and methods section

The section of materials and methods is actually process description. The complexity of scientific inquiry necessitates that the writing of materials and methods be clear and orderly to avoid confusion and ambiguity. It is crucial to clearly explain how you carried out your study step by step.

However, there is no set sequence for materials and methods section. Sub-headings are normally used to make a clear layout and good sub-headings make the paper skimmed easy and efficient. It is also a basic and effective method to write this section in chronological order and in order of importance.

8.3.1 Chronological order and order of importance

The content of materials and methods section and its subsections should be organized in a certain logical order, usually in chronological order or in order of importance. For example, independent variables are mentioned before dependent variables(先说明自变量再说明因变量). Firstly the determination of dependent variables are described to answer research questions before the determination of other dependent variables.

Besides，the use of subheadings and parentheses makes the description more coherent and consistent.

Briefly，the materials and methods section should be organized to make a clear and precise explanation according to the three questions：

- What was used?
- What was done?
- How was it done?

8.3.2　Subheadings and topic sentences

It is usually more effective to organize the materials and methods section under several different subheadings which are usually classified according to moves such as experimental design or procedures，materials，analytical techniques，or statistical analysis，etc. Taking advantages of the second and third level headings gives more hierarchy to the experimental materials and methods described in the section.

Take Sample 1 above as an example. This section is organized in six subheadings：
- Study design and participants，
- CT image acquisition，
- Image interpretation，
- Follow-up chest CT，
- Statistical analysis，
- Role of the funding source.

Though the skeletons of materials and methods section may vary in journal articles，the "moves" in this section generally involve working through a series of subsections with sub-headings，including measures，procedures，participants，analytical techniques，or statistical analysis. Normally，if no participants are involved，the method simply describes the measures and procedure(s) (Hartley，2008). When possible，you should construct sub-headings that match those to be used in results.

Besides，the materials and methods section could also be divided into several subsections by beginning with a topic sentence in each subsection to indicate the main topic or message of the paragraph.

8.3.3　Tenses

The use of tenses in materials and methods section depends on specific situations.

In most cases，the verb tense in materials and methods section is the past tense partly because it is a description of completed action，partly because of convention.

For example, when describing selected samples, designed materials or equipment, the past tense is usually used.

However, present tense is also used when describing how data are presented in the paper, when describing general population from which the samples are taken, and when presenting conventional materials or equipment.

Passive voice is often preferred in lab reports and scientific research papers because this section generally focuses on experimental procedures and the materials used rather than the person who conducted the study.

[**Sample 2**]

1) Here we provide a system-level analysis of the multi-sided ecology(多重生态) of nearly 100 million individuals expressing views regarding vaccination, which are emerging from the approximately 3 billion users of Facebook from across countries, continents and languages.

2) Images from cases seen at Wuhan Jinyintan Hospital were interpreted by two radiologists experienced in thoracic radiology (YF [12 years' experience] and NJ [10 years' experience]). All Digital Imaging and Communications in Medicine (DICOM) images from the CT studies were analyzed without access to clinical or laboratory findings.

3) The Department of Conversation and National Resources and the state Department of Environmental Protection has been investigating the course of the outbreak and testing the entire infrastructure at Cowans Gap, including the sewage system and widespread testing of the lake.

4) The trial protocol with the statistical analysis plan is available at NEJM. org. The trial was designed and overseen by representatives of the trial sponsor (Novo Nordisk) with input from selected site investigators.

8.4 Moves in the materials and methods section

Materials and methods are usually integrated and could also be introduced separately in some papers which mainly explain the procedural steps and materials used in the study.

In the materials and methods section, you should fully and exactly describe the new or improved techniques employed in your research. If the techniques have already been described by others, then it is adequate and desirable to refer to the paper where the technique was first described.

The main moves or basic elements are included in the following table.

Table 8 - 1　Main moves or basic elements

Moves	Content
Overview	A brief summary of the study method
Sites or places	A description of the location/condition of the research including inclusion criteria or sampling methods
Participants or materials	A description of the sampling methods, participants involved (groups of people related to age, sex, etc.) or animals selected
Methods, measurement or detection techniques	Methods, instruments and reagents/kits used for measuring or detecting the samples collected
Limitations	An indication of the limitations or restrictions of the method
Variables	A description of changing factors in the experiment
Procedures	A description of detailed processes to obtain the data
Data analysis	A description of methods used to analyze the data (statistical methods, computer or mathematical models)

In many cases, experimental design is the principle of data collection covering all the elements of the materials and methods. Experimental design and data collection procedures must be integrated. When reading a paper, many researchers and scientists are always able to get sharp judgment on experimental design and data collection procedures.

A clear description of a well-done experimental design is essential. The hypothesis to be tested, independent variables and dependent variables must be included and taken into careful consideration.

Data analysis is to indicate what types of statistical methods and mathematical models were used to determine statistical significance, to get further results and to test the hypotheses. Without careful data analysis, the results of a scientific research compromise the reliability of the results.

[**Sample 3**]

HFRS(肾综合征出血热) is one of the Class B Notifiable Diseases, and data have been reported since 1950 according to a standard protocol. In this study, HFRS data from 1970 to 2010 was obtained from the China Notifiable Disease Reporting System (CNDRS). The cases analysed included clinical cases and laboratory confirmed cases. Clinical diagnosis criteria included: exposure history (i. e. direct or indirect exposure to rodents and their excreta and saliva within two months before the onset of illness); acute onset with at least two of the following clinical symptoms (i. e. fever $> 38\ ℃$, chills, haemorrhagic manifestations, headache, back pain, abdominal pain, acute renal dysfunction and hypotension); experience or partial experience of the five phases of disease course (i. e. fever, hypopiesis, oliguresis, hyperdiuresis and recovery) and abnormal blood and urine routine parameters. Laboratory-confirmed case diagnosis criteria were clinical diagnosis with one of the positive laboratory tests (HV anti-IgM positive, four-fold increasing of anti-IgG and virus isolated from serum or detected HV RNA).

All data recorded for HFRS cases from 1970 to 2010 were extracted for statistical analysis by time, region and profession; the incidence rate was obtained directly from CNDRS. We analyzed the morbidity and mortality data of HFRS from 2006 to 2010. This period was China's Eleventh Five-Year Plan, during which time much work was done to prevent and control communicable diseases including HFRS. In 2008, China began the expanded immunization programme for HFRS vaccine, which targeted susceptible people in high-endemic districts to control the HFRS incidence.

Data were organized in Microsoft Excel spreadsheets and processed with SPSS 13.0 software. (Huang et al., 2012)

[**Analysis**]

The scope and source of research data are explained in the first two sentences.

Then, the research participants and detailed inclusion criteria are described. Accordingly, sites or places, participants, and procedures are included in the first paragraph.

The second paragraph mainly describes the content and methods of statistical analysis, especially making clear the content and methods of key analysis.

Data analysis is mentioned in the last paragraph: "Data were organized in Microsoft Excel spreadsheets and processed with SPSS 13.0 software."

Chapter Review

In this chapter, we have discussed how to write the section of materials and methods that conforms to international norms, including functions conveyed in this section, principles to be observed, moves in materials and methods and its well-organized discourse. etc.

- Generally, the materials and methods section reports everything involved in the research process. There are at least 5 main moves or basic elements offering a framework for the research process and data analysis.
- Sufficient details must be provided in the materials and methods section in order to allow any of the related researchers to repeat the experiments with an equal likelihood of obtaining similar results.

Assignments

Task 1   *The following materials and methods section, with the subheadings missing, are extracted from an SCI paper.*

- *Read it through, and then choose the most appropriate subheading for each subsection from the given subheadings in the box.*
- *Then, discuss with your classmates and try to identify and understand how the author described the main moves or basic elements（Sites or places, Participants, Measurement or detection techniques, Procedures and Data analysis）.*

A. Materials
B. Statistical Analysis
C. Experimental Design
D. Estimating Lifetime Risk of Stroke
E. Statistical Modeling
F. Estimating Stroke Incidence and Mortality

Global, Regional, and Country-Specific Lifetime Risks of Stroke, 1990 and 2016

1. _____

We used estimates from the GBD Study 2016 of the rate of first stroke, cause-specific mortality, and all-cause mortality at the global, regional (21 GBD regions nested within 7 GBD superregions), and national (195 countries) levels, stratified according to age and sex. Analyses were performed separately for ischemic stroke and hemorrhagic stroke; the latter included intracerebral hemorrhagic stroke and nontraumatic subarachnoid hemorrhagic stroke. The GBD Study 2016 used all available representative population-based data on incidence, prevalence, case fatality, and mortality to produce estimates of disease burden in 195 countries according to sex and 5-year age categories. Mortality was estimated by means of the Cause of Death Ensemble model, in which vital registration, verbal autopsy data (which included a written summary of events leading to a person's death as well as answers to standardized questions obtained by trained workers from families or other reliable informants in the local language), and country-specific covariates are used to estimate cause-specific mortality over time. Stroke incidence was estimated with the use of DisMod-MR, a Bayesian meta-regression disease modeling tool. Details of the methods that we used to estimate stroke incidence and mortality have been previously published and are summarized in the Supplementary Appendix.

2. _____

Countries were categorized into quintiles of the SDI（high，high-medium，medium，medium-low，and low level of development）used in the GBD Study 2016. The SDI，a composite indicator of development similar to the Human Development Index，is based on country-level income per capita，average educational attainment among persons older than 15 years of age，and total fertility rate. We used stroke incidence，prevalence，and mortality rates in each 5-year age group to estimate the lifetime risk of stroke among persons at a given age. The lifetime risk of stroke at each age represents the cumulative risk of stroke from that age onward and is conditional on a person's survival to that age without having had a nonfatal stroke. Further details are provided in the Supplementary Appendix.

To account for the competing risks of stroke and death within a specific age group，we calculated the probability of both stroke and death from any cause other than stroke separately and then scaled the separate event probabilities to match the combined probability of both events. We calculated the lifetime risk only among persons 25 years of age or older because incidence rates of stroke among younger persons are low and are less dependent on modifiable risk factors and on the characteristics of health systems，which are associated with stroke burden in older populations.

3. _____

Point estimates and 95% uncertainty intervals representing the 2.5th and 97.5th percentiles around the estimate were used to compare results between groups. Differences in the estimates of the risk of stroke were considered to be significant when the 95% uncertainty intervals did not overlap or when the 95% uncertainty interval for relative percentage change did not include zero. (The GBD 2016；2018)

Task 2 *The following subsection is extracted from the materials and methods section of a SCI paper.*

- *Read it through and select the appropriate word or words to fill in the blanks.*
- *Then，discuss with your partners and try to identify and understand how the author presented and described the data sources and procedures.*

Exposure to paternal tobacco smoking increased child hospitalization for lower respiratory infections but not for other diseases in Vietnam

Data sources and procedures

We did a secondary analysis of the most recent（as at December，2015）Demographic and Health Survey（DHS）data from 28 LMICs where both tobacco use and HIV test data were made publicly available. Access to and use of this data ___1___（have been/was）authorised by the DHS programme. The DHS is designed to collect cross-sectional data that ___2___（are/were）nationally representative of the health and welfare of women of reproductive age（15—49 years），their children，and their households at about 5-year intervals across many LMICs. The DHS ___3___（program/procedure）including the two-staged ___4___（sampling/investigating）approach for the selection of census enumeration areas and households，questionnaire validation，data collection for household，men，and women，and data ___5___（validation/analysis）are comprehensively described elsewhere. In all selected households，women aged 15—49 years are eligible to participate，and those who give consent are ___6___（interviewed/exanimated）using a women's questionnaire. In many surveys，men aged 15—54 years（or up to 59 years in some instances）from a subsample of the main survey households are also eligible to participate，and those who give consent are interviewed using a men's questionnaire. The ___7___（results/surveys）are comparable across countries through the use of standard model questionnaires and sampling methods.

In the DHS，___8___（women/tobacco）use is ascertained by three questions to be answered "yes" or "no". Two are about whether the respondent currently smokes cigarettes or uses any other type of tobacco. The third asks the respondent what types of tobacco they currently smoke or use，for which all tobacco types are recorded including country-specific products. HIV status data are obtained from a HIV testing protocol that undergoes a host country ethical review and provides status from informed，anonymous，and ___9___（random/voluntary）HIV testing for both women and men. Blood spots are collected on filter paper from a finger prick and transported to a laboratory for testing. The testing ___10___（involves/involved）an initial ELISA test，and then retesting of all positive tests and 5%—10% of the negative tests with a second ELISA. For those with discordant results on the two ELISA tests，a new ELISA or a western blot is done.（Miyahara et al.，2018）

Task 3　*The following 12 sentences or paragraphs that have been disordered are from the materials and methods section of a paper on catheter ablation research*（导管消融术研究）. *Rearrange the following parts into an organized materials and methods section* *by numbering them from 1 to 12，focusing on functional keywords and context and ignoring unfamiliar words.*

_____ A. **Catheter ablation of AF**

Patients scheduled for AF ablation underwent MRI of the pulmonary veins （PV） and left atrium （LA） before the procedure to identify anatomical variants, to assess the exact anatomical position and size of PV ostia and to merge with CARTO 3 system （Biosense Webster, Diamond Bar, CA, USA）.

_____ B. A 6 F steerable decapolar Dynamic XT catheter （Boston Scientific, Marlborough, MA, USA） was positioned in the coronary sinus for mapping and pacing purposes. For ablation an 8 F Thermocool bi-directional （D-F curve） catheter was used （Biosense Webster, Diamond Bar, CA, USA）. A steerable 7 F multipolar Lasso catheter （Biosense Webster, Diamond Bar, CA, USA） was used for mapping of the PVs and to confirm procedural endpoint of electrical isolation.

_____ C. The procedural endpoint was electrical isolation （entrance and exit block） documented using the Lasso mapping catheter. Power was limited to 30 Watts and flow was adjusted from 2 mL/min up to 30 mL/min to achieve this power. In patients with a history of typical AFL （5 patients in our group） a cavo-tricuspid isthmus ablation line was added. If sinus rhythm was not restored following ablation, the patient was cardioverted with a direct current shock.

_____ D. Few patients with other tachyarrhythmias were also enrolled: 2 with typical atrial flutter （AFL）, 3 with idiopathic ventricular extrasystole （VES） from the right ventricular outflow tract （RVOT） and 1 with atrioventricular nodal reentry tachycardia （AVNRT）. Percutaneous access for all catheters was via the right femoral vein. Written informed consent was obtained from all patients. All clinical cardiac characteristics as well as important comorbidities were recorded according to the regulations of the local Institutional Committee on Human Research. This was a single-center study.

_____ E. Catheter positioning into and within the cardiac chamber of interest as well as mapping and ablation were attempted without fluoroscopy with the support of EMA. A fast anatomical map was created using the Lasso catheter to create a 3D geometry of LA and PV without fluoroscopy. PV isolation was performed by wide-area circumferential point-bypoint RFA around the ostia of the ipsilateral PVs.

_____ F. Among patients referred to the Division of Arrhythmia and Electrophysiology at the University Heart Center in Zurich, Switzerland, 34 patients were enrolled consecutively in the study. Majority of patients in the study group were referred for RFA of AF (28 patients).

_____G. TEE was also done before the procedure to rule out thrombi in the LA and to document the presence of a patent foramen ovale (PFO). For mapping and ablation, a 3D EAM system, CARTO 3 system (Biosense Webster, Diamond Bar, CA, USA) was used. All procedures were performed under conscious sedation using midazolam and fentanyl.

_____H. Procedural safety pre-procedure and post-procedure patient management, as well as intra-procedure anticoagulation policy were in accordance with practice guidelines and our hospital policies.

_____I. All operators performing the ablation procedures were senior staff with experience in catheter navigation under 3D EAM system. Different imaging modalities were used including intracardiac echocardiography (ICE), transesophageal echocardiography (TEE) and magnetic resonance imaging (MRI) as needed. Although the intention was to perform zero fluoroscopy procedure, all operators were allowed to use fluoroscopy if required for patient safety and that is why fluoroscopy was used in 13 patients.

_____J. In 5 patients the catheters were introduced to LA through a PFO without the need of TSP. In 3 patients with PFO, ICE was used to allocate the site of PFO that was crossed by the ablation catheter along with its Preface guiding sheath.

_____K. The transseptal punctures (TSP) were performed using Brockenborough (BRK-1) needle (St. Jude Medical, St. Paul, MN, USA) through 8 F Preface guiding sheath (Biosense Webster, Diamond Bar, CA, USA) and was attempted under the guidance of Acuson Acuna ultrasound catheter (Siemens Healthcare, Erlangen, Germany).

_____L. In 2 patients with PFO, the ablation catheter (through the Preface guiding sheath) was brought to the superior vena cava and dragged caudally till the typical jump to the foramen ovale region was detected with 3D EAM. Then the ablation catheter along with its guiding sheath were advanced into the LA. (Haegeli et al., 2019)

Task 4　*Now work with your partner to identify the headings and subheadings in the following articles in Appendix Ⅱ through scanning the QR code below. Answer the following questions:*

1. Why are there variations in headings and subheadings?
2. Why is it necessary to organize information under different subheadings?
3. What information do the subheadings convey?

Appendix	Title	Headings	Subheadings
1	Observational Study of Hydroxychloroquine ...		
3	Genetic Modification and Screening ...		
5	Early Prediction of Circulatory Failure ...		
7	Radiological Findings from 81 Patients with COVID-19 ...		

Task 5　*Complete the following sentences by translating the expression in parentheses into English.*

1. The experimental study was done on 20 cases of _____ _____（提供了知情同意书的健康志愿受试者）.

2. The sensitivity analysis _____（进一步确定了）the most important parameters that drive each of the systems in Table 2.

3. We screened a random sample of 1,200 subjects of all age groups selected by clustering. _____ （确定了主要的和次要的诊断标准），and a severity score was developed and applied.

4. _____（对分离病毒进行的基因测序显示）that they are linked to WPV3（野生 3 型脊灰病毒）detected in mid-2008 in northern Nigeria.

5. In its simplest and most basic form, steganalysis is performed _____ _____（通过使用统计分析技术）.

6. _____ _____（确保数据完整性）by verifying that all participants in the replicate have table and replicated column attributes that match the master replicate definition.

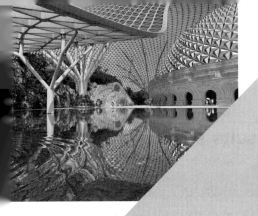

Chapter Nine

Results Writing

Lead-in Questions

1. Which is probably the most important part of an academic paper?
2. What is the function of the results section?
3. What is the basic structure of the results section?

Learning Objectives

After learning this unit, you will be able to:

1. present the findings in a logical and orderly way,
2. organize the results with proper items,
3. and choose descriptive words precisely.

✓参考答案
✓课件申请
✓学术资源

9.1 The function of the results section

The hypothesis of a study has been proposed in the introduction and the collected supporting data have been provided in the materials and methods section. The problem is that the data provided by the methods are just raw data, and these raw data are far from enough to prove the validity of the hypothesis. At this point, there must be an effective means to link the hypothesis with the data, which makes the data meaningful to prove whether the hypothesis is true or not. It is the results section that undertakes this task by translating the raw data into meaningful results without interpretation. Therefore, the function of the results section is to objectively report the key findings in the research in an orderly and logical sequence, that is, to state the results of the experiments described in the materials and methods section. In addition, the results section directs the readers to figures or tables that present supporting data.

More specifically, according to Swales & Feak (2012), some of the common functions of the results section should be:

- highlighting the results of research,
- using data to support a point or make an argument in the paper,
- assessing theory, common beliefs, or general practice in light of the given data,
- comparing and evaluating different data sets,
- assessing the reliability of the data in terms of the methodology that produced it,
- discussing the implications of the data,
- and making recommendations.

Actually, not all of the above items are obliged to be included in the results section, but some of the essential items should be included.

9.2 The items and organization of the results section

9.2.1 Items

It's not an easy job to describe an exact structural framework on how to write the results section in an academic paper. It would be helpful to start with the items below which should usually be included in the results section, and some of the common rules below, so that you could get a rough notion about how to write results.

Table 9 - 1 Rules for constructing results

Items included in results section	Rules for writing results section
comparison of two or more measurements	when comparing results, avoid ambiguous interpretations
statistical graphs including tables, figures, diagrams and charts	to use tables, figures, diagrams and charts to report the results
report of general tendency in data	if numbers are better in explanation, use less textual explanation
summary of important points from statistical graphs	the text around tables/figures/diagrams/charts should give a thorough exposition
important findings observed from the experiment or research	to list the results according to their importance
subheadings	to label the tables, figures, diagrams and charts and give each of them a short title
summary of main findings	arrange in an appropriate logical order

In the results section, the key findings of the research should be presented in an orderly and logical sequence by using text and illustrative materials such as tables, figures and charts.

9.2.2 Organization

For hypothesis-testing studies in which all the experiments are designed in advance, organize the results section either chronologically or from most to least importance. Present your results in logical sequence in the text, tables, and illustrations, with the main or most important findings first. Do not repeat all the data in the tables or illustrations in the text.

For hypothesis-testing studies in which one experiment determines what the next experiment will be, the results section is organized in a repeating four-part pattern: question, overview of the experiments, results, answer to the question. If necessary, background indicating why the question was asked and purposes and reasons explaining why the experiment was done are also included.

Extra or supplementary materials and technical details can be placed in an appendix where they will be accessible but will not interrupt the flow of the text.

9.2.3 Length

Many authors try to put the whole paper into the results section—methods, figure legends, table titles, results, data, comparisons with the literature—in fact, everything except the introduction. This temptation should be resisted. The results section should be as brief and uncluttered as possible so that the readers can see the forest for the trees.

9.3 The structure of data commentary

Data are used when describing trends or directions, and figures used when specific magnitudes are required. In many academic papers, the findings usually provide three elements of information(Weissberg & Buker, 1990; Swales & Feak, 2012):

- **Location elements**: locating the figure(s) where the results come;
- **Highlighting elements**: presenting the key findings, generalizing the data; (central part of a data commentary)
- **Commenting elements**: commenting on the results, interpretation or implication of the results.

[**Sample 1**]

(1) From 1970 to 2010, 1 546 063 HFRS cases were recorded. (2) The annual HFRS incidence rose <u>steadily</u> in the early 1970s but experienced an <u>alarming</u> increase in the early 1980s. (3) Case numbers <u>peaked</u> in 1986, when 115 804 cases were reported in Mainland China. From 1987 to 2010, however, HFRS case numbers decreased, with <u>occasional small fluctuations</u>. (4) Eventually, in 2009, HFRS case numbers reached its <u>lowest</u> number (8 745) since 1986, followed by a <u>slight</u> rise in 2010 (9 526) (Figure 1). (Huang et al., 2012)

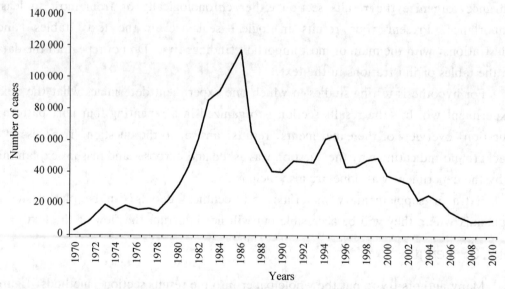

Figure 1　Annual haemorrhagic fever with renal syndrome incidence in Mainland China from 1970 to 2010

[**Analysis**]

The data and figure in Sample 1 show the trends and the specific magnitudes of SHFR. The first sentence is location statement and sentences 2, 3 & 4 are highlighting statements.

Yet, interpretation and implication are not presented in this paragraph.

By the way, in this paragraph we can see some smart words and phrases: steadily, alarming, peak, occasional small fluctuations, lowest and slight. These words and phrases express and provide the magnitude, trend or degree reflected by the data and figure. They make the trends and magnitudes more vivid and accurate.

9.4   The writing requirements of the results section

9.4.1   The writing style

Given the characteristics of the results, the writing style should be calm, clear, explicit and objective. The message of the topic sentences should be given as results, instead of a method. The results section usually begins with text.

9.4.2   Tense and voice of the results section

Results of hypothesis-testing studies and of tests of new methods in methods papers are reported in the past tense, because they are discrete events that occurred in the past. Meanwhile, when describing specific results and referring to a figure or table, different verb tense-voice could be used in combination depending on the situation.

Table 9 - 2   Different verb tense-voice combinations

Function	Tense-voice combination	Examples
To describe specific results	Past-active	PrPc did not alter the expression levels of MMP2 and MMP9 proteins.
	Past-passive	The expression levels of phosphorylated p38 MAPKs, phosphorylated JNKs and total ERK protein were not altered.
To refer to a figure or a table	Present-active	Figure 1 shows the mass spectrum of the PFBOA derivative of methional.
	Present-passive	The values of OD in different groups are shown in Tab 1

Therefore, the tenses used in the results can be summarized as follows:

• Past simple tense. Results should be reported in the past simple tense because results are discrete events that have occured. Since the research has been done, when it is reported and explained in the results section, it is appropriate to use the past simple tense rather than the present simple tense.

• Passive voice. In an academic paper, the passive voice is used more frequently because it is inappropriate and impolite to always use active voice emphasizing the author's contribution. However, active voice can still be used when the circumstance allows.

9.4.3 Identifying human subjects

Do not use initials to identify study subjects. Use A, B, C, etc., if you refer to an individual subject. Use 1, 2, 3, etc., when you studied more than 26 subjects.

9.4.4 Comparisons

When comparing results, avoid ambiguous statements such as "A was increased compared with B." Instead write "A was greater than B", "A increased more than B" or "A increased but B was unchanged."

Also, avoid ambiguous statements such as "showed some promising trends."

9.4.5 Statistics

Given numeric results not only as derivatives (for example, percentages) but also as the absolute numbers from which the derivatives were calculated, and specify the statistical methods used to analyze them.

Here is an example from a recently published article on the study of clinical characteristics of COVID-19 which outbroke in Wuhan and rapidly spread throughout China. The authors collected data from 1 099 confirmed patients from 552 hospitals in mainland China. The primary composite end point was admission to an intensive care unit (ICU), the use of mechanical ventilation, or death.

Sample 2 is a good example to contrast and reflect on all the requirements above.

[Sample 2]
Results
Demographic and Clinical Characteristics

Of the 7 736 patients with COVID-19 who had been hospitalized at 552 sites as of January 29, 2020 we obtained data regarding clinical symptoms and outcomes for 1 099 patients (14.2%). The largest number of patients (132) had been admitted to Wuhan Jinyintan Hospital. The hospitals that were included in this study accounted or 29.7% of the 1 856 designated hospitals where patients with COVID-19 could be admitted in 30 provinces, autonomous regions, or municipalities across China.

The demographic and clinical characteristics of the patients are shown in Table 1. A total of 3.5% were health care workers, and a history of contact with wildlife was documented in 1.9%; 483 patients (43.9%) were residents of Wuhan. Among the patients who lived outside Wuhan, 72.3% had contact with residents of Wuhan, including 31.3% who had visited the city; 25.9% of nonresidents had neither visited the city nor had contact with Wuhan residents.

Table 1. Clinical Characteristics of the Study Patients, According to Disease Severity and the Presence or Absence of the Primary Composite End Point. *

Characteristics	All Patients (N = 1 099)	Disease Severity		Presence of Primary Composite End Point†	
		Nonsevere (N = 926)	Severe (N = 173)	Yes (N = 67)	No (N = 1 032)
Age					
Median(IQR)—yr	47.0 (35.0~58.0)	45.0 (34.0~57.0)	52.0 (40.0~65.0)	63.0 (53.0~71.0)	46.0 (35.0~57.0)
Distribution—no./total no. (%)					
0~14 yr	9/1 011(0.9)	8/848(0.9)	1/163(0.6)	0	9/946(1.0)
15~49 yr	557/1 011 (55.1)	490/848 (57.8)	67/163 (41.1)	12/65 (18.5)	545/946 (57.6)
50~64 yr	292/1 011 (28.9)	241/848 (28.4)	51/163 (31.3)	21/65 (32.3)	271/946 (28.6)
≥65 yr	153/1 011 (15.1)	109/848 (12.9)	44/163 (27.0)	32/65 (49.2)	121/946 (12.8)
Female sex—no./total no. (%)	459/1 096 (41.9)	386/923 (41.8)	73/173 (42.2)	22/67 (32.8)	437/1 029 (42.5)
Smoking history—no./total no. (%)					
Never smoked	927/1 085 (85.4)	793/913 (86.9)	134/172 (77.9)	44/66 (66.7)	883/1 019 (86.7)
Former smoker	21/1 085 (1.9)	12/913 (1.3)	9/172 (5.2)	5/66 (7.6)	16/1 019 (1.6)
Current smoker	137/1 085 (12.6)	108/913 (11.8)	29/172 (16.9)	17/66 (25.8)	120/1 019 (11.8)
Exposure to source of transmission within past 14 days—no./total no.					
Living in Wuhan	483/1 099 (43.9)	400/926 (43.2)	83/173 (48.0)	39/67 (58.2)	444/1 032 (43.0)
Contact with wildlife	13/687 (1.9)	10/559 (1.8)	3/128 (2.3)	1/41 (2.4)	12/646 (1.9)
Recently visited Wuhan‡	193/616 (31.3)	166/526 (31.6)	27/90 (30.0)	10/28 (35.7)	183/588 (31.1)
Had contact with Wuhan residents‡	442/611 (72.3)	376/522 (72.0)	66/89 (74.2)	19/28 (67.9)	423/583 (72.6)

(Continued)

Characteristics	All Patients (N = 1 099)	Disease Severity		Presence of Primary Composite End Point†	
		Nonsevere (N = 926)	Severe (N = 173)	Yes (N = 67)	No (N = 1 032)
Median incubation period (IQR)—days §	4.0 (2.0～7.0)	4.0 (2.8～7.0)	4.0 (2.0～7.0)	4.0 (1.0～7.5)	4.0 (2.0～7.0)
Fever on admission					
Patients—no./tatal no.(%)	473/1 081 (43.8)	391/910 (43.0)	82/171 (48.0)	24/66 (36.4)	449/1 015 (44.2)
Median temperature (IQR)—℃	37.3 (36.7～38.0)	37.3 (36.7～38.0)	37.4 (36.7～38.1)	36.8 (36.3～37.8)	37.3 (36.7～38.0)
Distribution of temperature—no./total no.(%)					
<37.5℃	608/1 081 (56.2)	519/910 (57.0)	89/171 (52.0)	42/66 (63.6)	566/1 015 (55.8)
37.5～38.0℃	238/1 081 (22.0)	201/910 (22.1)	37/171 (21.6)	10/66 (15.2)	228/1 015 (22.5)
38.1～39.0℃	197/1 081 (18.2)	160/910 (17.6)	37/171 (21.6)	11/66 (16.7)	186/1 015 (18.3)
>39.0℃	38/1 081 (3.5)	30/910 (3.3)	8/171 (4.7)	3/66 (4.5)	35/1 015 (3.4)
Fever during hospitalization					
Patients—no./total no.(%)	975/1 099 (88.7)	816/926 (88.1)	159/173 (91.9)	59/67 (88.1)	916/1 032 (88.8)
Median highest temperature(IQR)—℃	38.3 (37.8～38.9)	38.3 (37.8～38.9)	38.5 (38.0～39.0)	38.5 (38.0～39.0)	38.3 (37.8～38.9)
<37.5℃	92/926 (9.9)	79/774 (10.2)	13/152 (8.6)	3/54 (5.6)	89/872 (10.2)
37.5～38.0℃	286/926 (30.9)	251/774 (32.4)	35/152 (23.0)	20/54 (37.0)	266/872 (30.5)
38.1～39.0℃	434/926 (46.9)	356/774 (46.0)	78/152 (51.3)	21/54 (38.9)	413/872 (47.4)
>39.0℃	114/926 (12.3)	88/774 (11.4)	26/152 (17.1)	10/54 (18.5)	104/872 (11.9)
Symptoms—no.(%)					
Conjunctival congestion	9(0.8)	5(0.5)	4(2.3)	0	9(0.9)
Nasal congestion	53(4.8)	47(5.1)	6(3.5)	2(3.0)	51(4.9)
Headache	150(13.6)	124(13.4)	26(15.0)	8(11.9)	142(13.8)
Cough	745(67.8)	623(67.3)	122(70.5)	46(68.7)	699(67.7)

(Continued)

Characteristics	All Patients (N = 1 099)	Disease Severity		Presence of Primary Composite End Point†	
		Nonsevere (N = 926)	Severe (N = 173)	Yes (N = 67)	No (N = 1 032)
Sore throat	153(13.9)	130(14.0)	23(13.3)	6(9.0)	147(14.2)
Sputum production	370(33.7)	309(33.4)	61(35.3)	20(29.9)	350(33.9)
Fatigue	419(38.1)	350(37.8)	69(39.9)	22(32.8)	397(38.5)
Hemoptysis	10(0.9)	6(0.6)	4(2.3)	2(3.0)	8(0.8)
Shortness of breath	205(18.7)	140(15.1)	65(37.6)	36(53.7)	169(16.4)
Nausea or vomiting	55(5.0)	43(4.6)	12(6.9)	3(4.5)	52(5.0)
Diarrhea	42(3.8)	32(3.5)	10(5.8)	4(6.0)	38(3.7)
Myalgia or arthralgia	164(14.9)	134(14.5)	30(17.3)	6(9.0)	158(15.3)
Chills	126(11.5)	100(10.8)	26(15.0)	8(11.9)	118(11.4)
Signs of infection—no. (%)					
Throat congestion	19(1.7)	17(1.8)	2(1.2)	0	19(1.8)
Tonsil swelling	23(2.1)	17(1.8)	6(3.5)	1(1.5)	22(2.1)
Enlargement of lymph nodes	2(0.2)	1(0.1)	1(0.6)	1(1.5)	1(0.1)
Rash	2(0.2)	0	2(1.2)	0	2(0.2)
Coexisting disorder—no. (%)					
Any	261(23.7)	194(21.0)	67(38.7)	39(58.2)	222(21.5)
Chronic obstructive pulmonary disease	12(1.1)	6(0.6)	6(3.5)	7(10.4)	5(0.5)
Diabetes	81(7.4)	53(5.7)	28(16.2)	18(26.9)	63(6.1)
Hypertension	165(15.0)	124(13.4)	41(23.7)	24(35.8)	141(13.7)
Coronary heart disease	27(2.5)	17(1.8)	10(5.8)	6(9.0)	21(2.0)
Cerebrovascular disease	15(1.4)	11(1.2)	4(2.3)	4(6.0)	11(1.1)
Hepatitis B infection¶	23(2.1)	22(2.4)	1(0.6)	1(1.5)	22(2.1)
Cancer ‖	10(0.9)	7(0.8)	3(1.7)	1(1.5)	9(0.9)
Chronic renal disease	8(0.7)	5(0.5)	3(1.7)	2(3.0)	6(0.6)
Immunodeficiency	2(0.2)	2(0.2)	0	0	2(0.2)

* The denominators of patients who were included in the analysis are provided if they differed from the overall numbers in the group. Percentages may not total 100 because of rounding. COVID-19 denotes coronavirus disease 2019, and IQR interquartile range.

† The primary composite end point was admission to an intensive care unit, the use of mechanical ventilation, or death.

‡ These patients were not residents of Wuhan.

§ Data regarding the incubation period were missing for 808 patients(73.5%).

¶ The presence of hepatitis B infection was defined as a positive result on testing for hepatitis B surface antigen with or without elevated levels of alanine or aspartate aminotransferase.

‖ Included in this category is any type of cancer.

The median incubation period was 4 days (interquartile range, 2 to 7). The median age of the patients was 47 years (interquartile range, 35 to 58); 0.9% of the patients were younger than 15 years of age. A total of 41.9% were female. Fever was present in 43.8% of the patients on admission but developed in 88.7% during hospitalization. The second most common symptom was cough (67.8%); nausea or vomiting (5.0%) and diarrhea (3.8%) were uncommon. Among the overall population, 23.7% had at least one coexisting illness (e. g., hypertension and chronic obstructive pulmonary disease).

On admission, the degree of severity of COVID-19 was categorized as non-severe in 926 patients and severe in 173 patients. Patients with severe disease were older than those with non-severe disease by a median of 7 years. Moreover, the presence of any coexisting illness was more common among patients with severe disease than among those with non-severe disease (38.7% vs. 21.0%). However, the exposure history between the two groups of disease severity was similar.

Radiologic and Laboratory Findings

Table 2 shows the radiologic and laboratory findings on admission. Of 975 CT scans that were performed at the time of admission, 86.2% revealed abnormal results. The most common patterns on chest CT were ground-glass opacity (56.4%) and bilateral patchy shadowing (51.8%). Representative radiologic findings in two patients with non-severe COVID-19 and in another two patients with severe COVID-19 are provided in Figure S1 in the Supplementary Appendix. No radiographic or CT abnormality was found in 157 of 877 patients (17.9%) with non-severe disease and in 5 of 173 patients (2.9%) with severe disease.

Table 2. Radiographic and Laboratory Findings*

Variables	All Patients (N = 1 099)	Disease Severity		Presence of Composite Primary End Point	
		Nonsevere (N = 926)	Severe (N = 173)	Yes (N = 67)	No (N = 1 032)
Radiologic findings					
Abnormalities on chest radiograph—no./total no.(%)	162/274 (59.1)	116/214 (54.2)	46/60 (76.7)	30/39 (76.9)	132/235 (56.2)

(Continued)

Variables	All Patients (N=1 099)	Disease Severity		Presence of Composite Primary End Point	
		Nonsevere (N=926)	Severe (N=173)	Yes (N=67)	No (N=1 032)
Ground-glass opacity	55/274 (20.1)	37/214 (17.3)	18/60 (30.0)	9/39 (23.1)	46/235 (19.6)
Local patchy shadowing	77/274 (28.1)	56/214 (26.2)	21/60 (35.0)	13/39 (33.3)	64/235 (27.2)
Bilateral patchy shadowing	100/274 (36.5)	65/214 (30.4)	35/60 (58.3)	27/39 (69.2)	73/235 (31.1)
Interstitial abnormalities	12/274 (4.4)	7/214 (3.3)	5/60 (8.3)	6/39 (15.4)	6/235 (2.6)
Abnormalities on chest CT—no./total no.(%)	840/975 (86.2)	682/808 (84.4)	158/167 (94.6)	50/57 (87.7)	790/918 (86.1)
Ground-glass opacity	550/975 (56.4)	449/808 (55.6)	101/167 (60.5)	30/57 (52.6)	520/918 (56.6)
Local patchy shadowing	409/975 (41.9)	317/808 (39.2)	92/167 (55.1)	22/57 (38.6)	387/918 (42.2)
Bilateral patchy shadowing	505/975 (51.8)	368/808 (45.5)	137/167 (82.0)	40/57 (70.2)	465/918 (50.7)
Interstitial abnormalities	143/975 (14.7)	99/808 (12.3)	44/167 (26.3)	15/57 (26.3)	128/918 (13.9)
Laboratory findings					
Median Pao_2 : Flo_2 ratio (IQR)†	3.9 (2.9~4.7)	3.9 (2.9~4.5)	4.0 (2.8~5.2)	2.9 (2.2~5.4)	4.0 (3.1~4.6)
White-cell count Median (IQR)—per mm^3	4 700(3 500~ 6 000)	4 900(3 800~ 6 000)	3 700(3 000~ 6 200)	6 100(4 900~ 11 100)	4 700(3 500~ 5 900)
Distribution—no./total no.(%)					
>10 000 per mm^3	58/978 (5.9)	39/811 (4.8)	19/167 (11.4)	15/58 (25.9)	43/920 (4.7)
<4 000 per mm^3	330/978 (33.7)	228/811 (28.1)	102/167 (61.1)	8/58 (13.8)	322/920 (35.0)
Lymphocyte count					
Median(IQR)—per mm^3	1 000 (700~1 300)	1 000 (800~1 400)	800 (600~1 000)	700 (600~900)	1 000 (700~1 300)
Distribution—no./total no.(%)					
<1 500 per mm^3	731/879 (83.2)	584/726 (80.4)	147/153 (96.1)	50/54 (92.6)	681/825 (82.5)
Platelet count Median (IQR)—per mm^3	168 000 (132 000~ 207 000)	172 000 (139 000~ 212 000)	137 500 (99 000~ 179 500)	156 500 (114 200~ 195 000)	169 000 (133 000~ 207 000)

(**Continued**)

Variables	All Patients (N=1 099)	Disease Severity		Presence of Composite Primary End Point	
		Nonsevere (N=926)	Severe (N=173)	Yes (N=67)	No (N=1 032)
Distribution—no./total no.(%)					
<150 000 per mm³	315/869 (36.2)	225/713 (31.6)	90/156 (57.7)	27/58 (46.6)	288/811 (35.5)
Median hemoglobin (IQR)—g/dl‡	13.4 (11.9~14.8)	13.5 (12.0~14.8)	12.8 (11.2~14.1)	12.5 (10.5~14.0)	13.4 (12.0~14.8)
Distribution of other findings—no./total no.(%)					
C-reactive protein≥10 mg/liter	481/793 (60.7)	371/658 (56.4)	110/135 (81.5)	41/45 (91.1)	440/748 (58.8)
Procalcitonin≥0.5 ng/ml	35/633 (5.5)	19/516 (3.7)	16/117 (13.7)	12/50 (24.0)	23/583 (3.9)
Lactate dehydrogenase≥250 U/liter	277/675 (41.0)	205/551 (37.2)	72/124 (58.1)	31/44 (70.5)	246/631 (39.0)
Aspartate aminotransferase>40 U/liter	168/757 (22.2)	112/615 (18.2)	56/142 (39.4)	26/52 (50.0)	142/705 (20.1)
Alanine aminotransferase>40 U/liter	158/741 (21.3)	120/606 (19.8)	38/135 (28.1)	20/49 (40.8)	138/692 (19.9)
Total bilirubin>17.1 μmol/liter	76/722 (10.5)	59/594 (9.9)	17/128 (13.3)	10/48 (20.8)	66/674 (9.8)
Creatine kinase≥200 U/liter	90/657 (13.7)	67536 (12.5)	23/121 (19.0)	12/46 (26.1)	78/611 (12.8)
Creatinine≥133 μmol/liter	12/752 (1.6)	6/614 (1.0)	6/138 (4.3)	5/52 (9.6)	7/700 (1.0)
D-dimer≥0.5 mg/liter	260/560 (46.4)	195/451 (43.2)	65/109 (59.6)	34/49 (69.4)	226/511 (44.2)
Minerals §					
Median sodium (IQR)—mmol/liter	138.2 (136.1~140.3)	138.4 (136.6~140.4)	138.0 (136.0~140.0)	138.3 (135.0~141.2)	138.2 (136.1~140.2)
Median potassium (IQR)—mmol/liter	3.8 (3.5~4.2)	3.9 (3.6~4.2)	3.8 (3.5~4.1)	3.9 (3.6~4.1)	3.8 (3.5~4.2)
Median chloride (IQR)—mmol/liter	102.9 (99.7~105.6)	102.7 (99.7~105.3)	103.1 (99.8~106.0)	103.8 (100.8~107.0)	102.8 (99.6~105.3)

* Lymphocytopenia was defined as lymphocyte count of less than 1 500 per cubic millimeter. Thrombocytopenia was defined as a platelet count of less than 150 000 per cubic millimeter. To convert the values for creatinine to milligrams per deciliter, divide by 88.4.

† Data regarding the ratio of the partial pressure of arterial oxygen to the fraction of inspired oxygen(Pao₂:

Flo$_2$) were missing for 894 patients(81.3%).

‡ Data regarding hemoglobin were missing for 226 patients(20.6%).

§ Data were missing for the measurement of sodium in 363 patients(33.0%), for potassium in 349 patients (31.8%), and for chloride in 392 patients(35.7%).

On admission, lymphocytopenia was present in 83.2% of the patients, thrombocytopenia in 36.2%, and leukopenia in 33.7%. Most of the patients had elevated levels of C-reactive protein; less common were elevated levels of alanine aminotransferase, aspartate aminotransferase, creatine kinase, and d-dimer. Patients with severe disease had more prominent laboratory abnormalities (including lymphocytopenia and leukopenia) than those with non-severe disease.

Clinical Outcomes

None of the 1099 patients were lost to follow-up during the study. A primary composite end-point event occurred in 67 patients (6.1%), including 5.0% who were admitted to the ICU, 2.3% who underwent invasive mechanical ventilation, and 1.4% who died (Table 3). Among the 173 patients with severe disease, a primary composite end-point event occurred in 43 patients (24.9%). Among all the patients, the cumulative risk of the composite end point was 3.6%; among those with severe disease, the cumulative risk was 20.6%.

Table 3. Complications, treatments, and clinical outcomes

Variables	All Patients (N=1 099)	Disease Severity		Presence of Composite Primary End Point	
		Nonsevere (N=926)	Severe (N=173)	Yes (N=67)	No (N=1 032)
Complications					
Septic shock—no.(%)	12(1.1)	1(0.1)	11(6.4)	9(13.4)	3(0.3)
Acute respiratory distress syndrome—no.(%)	37(3.4)	10(1.1)	27(15.6)	27(40.3)	10(1.0)
Acute kidney injury—no.(%)	6(0.5)	1(0.1)	5(2.9)	4(6.0)	2(0.2)
Disseminated intravascular coagulation—no.(%)	1(0.1)	0	1(0.6)	1(1.5)	0
Rhabdomyolysis—no.(%)	2(0.2)	2(0.2)	0	0	2(0.2)
Physician-diagnosed pneumonia—no./total no.(%)	972/1 067 (91.1)	800/894 (89.5)	172/173 (99.4)	63/66 (95.5)	909/1 001 (90.8)
Median time until development of pneumonia(IQR)—days*					
After initial COVID-19 diagnosis	0.0 (0.0~1.0)	0.0 (0.0~1.0)	0.0 (0.0~2.0)	0.0 (0.0~3.5)	0.0 (0.0~1.0)
After onset of COVID-19 symptoms	3.0 (1.0~6.0)	3.0 (1.0~6.0)	5.0 (2.0~7.0)	4.0 (0.0~7.0)	3.0 (1.0~6.0)

(**Continued**)

Variables	All Patients (N = 1 099)	Disease Severity		Presence of Composite Primary End Point	
		Nonsevere (N = 926)	Severe (N = 173)	Yes (N = 67)	No (N = 1 032)
Treatments					
Intravenous antibiotics—no. (%)	637(58.0)	498(53.8)	139(80.3)	60(89.6)	577(55.9)
Oseltamivir—no. (%)	393(35.8)	313(33.8)	80(46.2)	36(53.7)	357(34.6)
Antifungal medication—no. (%)	31(2.8)	18(1.9)	13(7.5)	8(11.9)	23(2.2)
Systemic glucocorticoids—no. (%)	204(18.6)	127(13.7)	77(44.5)	35(52.2)	169(16.4)
Oxygen therapy—no. (%)	454(41.3)	331(35.7)	123(71.1)	59(88.1)	395(38.3)
Mechanical ventilation—no. (%)	67(6.1)	0	67(38.7)	40(59.7)	27(2.6)
Invasive	25(2.3)	0	25(14.5)	25(37.3)	0
Noninvasive	56(5.1)	0	56(32.4)	29(43.3)	27(2.6)
Use of extracorporeal membrane oxygenation—no. (%)	5(0.5)	0	5(2.9)	5(7.5)	0
Use of continuous renal-replacement therapy—no. (%)	9(0.8)	0	9(5.2)	8(11.9)	1(0.1)
Use of intravenous immune globulin—no. (%)	144(13.1)	86(9.3)	58(33.5)	27(40.3)	117(11.3)
Admission to intensive care unit—no. (%)	55(5.0)	22(2.4)	33(19.1)	55(82.1)	0
Median length of hospital stay(IQR)—days†	12.0 (10.0~14.0)	11.0 (10.0~13.0)	13.0 (11.5~17.0)	14.5 (11.0~19.0)	12.0 (10.0~13.0)
Clinical outcomes at data cutoff—no. (%)					
Discharge from hospital	55(5.0)	50(5.4)	5(2.9)	1(1.5)	54(5.2)
Death	15(1.4)	1(0.1)	14(8.1)	15(22.4)	0
Recovery	9(0.8)	7(0.8)	2(1.2)	0	9(0.9)
Hospitalization	1 029(93.6)	875(94.5)	154(89.0)	51(76.1)	978(94.8)

* For the development of pneumonia，data were missing for 347 patients(31.6%) regarding the time since the initial diagnosis and for 161 patients(14.6%) regarding the time since symptom onset.

† Data regarding the median length of hospital stay were missing for 136 patients(12.4%).

Treatment and Complications

A majority of the patients (58. 0%) received intravenous antibiotic therapy, and 35. 8% received oseltamivir therapy; oxygen therapy was administered in 41. 3% and mechanical ventilation in 6. 1%; higher percentages of patients with severe disease received these therapies (Table 3). Mechanical ventilation was initiated in more patients with severe disease than in those with non-severe disease (noninvasive ventilation, 32. 4% vs. 0%; invasive ventilation, 14. 5% vs. 0%). Systemic glucocorticoids were given to 204 patients (18. 6%), with a higher percentage among those with severe disease than nonsevere disease (44. 5% vs. 13. 7%). Of these 204 patients, 33 (16. 2%) were admitted to the ICU, 17 (8. 3%) underwent invasive ventilation, and 5 (2. 5%) died. Extracorporeal membrane oxygenation was performed in 5 patients (0. 5%) with severe disease.

The median duration of hospitalization was 12. 0 days (mean, 12. 8). During hospital admission, most of the patients received a diagnosis of pneumonia from a physician (91. 1%), followed by ARDS (3. 4%) and shock (1. 1%). Patients with severe disease had a higher incidence of physician-diagnosed pneumonia than those with non-severe disease (99. 4% vs. 89. 5%). (Guan et al. , 2020)

9.4.6 Precise word choice

1. Note the difference between ability and actuality.

• **Ability**: We could not demonstrate high-affinity, low-capacity DHE binding sites in heart particulates prepared from three adult sheep.

• **Actuality**: There were no high-affinity, low-capacity DHE binding sites in heart particulates prepared from three adult sheep.

"Could not demonstrate" implies that binding sites may have been there, but the technique was not sensitive enough to detect them. "There were no" implies that no binding sites exist (so no method would be able to detect them). Find out whether you are talking about ability or actuality, and choose your verb accordingly.

2. Note the difference between qualitative and quantitative statements.

Qualitative words that describe magnitude are imprecise and therefore of little value when used alone. Whenever possible, use quantitative rather than qualitative descriptions.

[**Sample 3**]

"Heart rate increased markedly. "

[**Analysis**]

What does "markedly" mean? We need the data to be sure how big the increase was. If you use a qualitative word such as "markedly," go on to quantify it, either by citing a figure or a table or by reporting the data (preferably as percent change) in the text. Write instead:

"Heart rate increased by 10%."

[Sample 4]

"Development rate was faster in the higher temperature treatment."

[Analysis]

What does "faster" imply? We also need the data to know how much "faster" and "faster" than what. Write instead: "Development rate in the 30 ℃ temperature treatment was 10% faster than that in the 20 ℃ temperature treatment."

Actually, the best policy is to avoid qualitative words altogether in the results section. Save qualitative words for the discussion, for occasions when you need to emphasize the magnitude of a change or a difference.

9.5 The content of the results section

9.5.1 What to be included in the results section

The primary information in the results section is results. However, not every result that you obtained from your experiments or observations needs to be reported in the results section. The results section should report only results pertinent to the question posed in the introduction. Results should be included whether or not they support your hypothesis. Both experimental and control results should be included.

In addition to presenting results, the results section can include a few data. However, most data, and in particular the most important data, should be presented in figures or tables, where the data are highly visible and easy to read. If a lot of data are presented in the text, they can overwhelm the results. Therefore, data should be kept to an absolute minimum in the results section. Data that are presented in a figure or a table should be omitted from the text. However, one or two especially important values can be repeated in the text for emphasis. In addition, brief secondary data that do not warrant display in a figure or a table can be presented in the text by being placed within parentheses after the result.

Normally, the results section does not include statements that need to be referenced, such as comparisons with others' results. However, if a brief comparison (one or two sentences) would not fit smoothly into the discussion, it can be included in the results section.

9.5.2 Results and data

Results are different from data. Data are facts, often numbers, obtained from experiments and observations. Data can be raw (for example, all the phospholipid concentrations measured during an experiment), summarized (for example, mean and SD), or transformed (for example, percent of control). Results are general statements that interpret data (for example, "Propranolol given during normal ventilation decreased phospholipid concentrations").

Data can rarely stand alone. The result (the meaning of the data) must be stated. See the example below.

[**Sample 5**]

In the 20 control subjects, the mean resting blood pressure was 85 ± 5 (SD) mmHg. In comparison, in the 30 tennis players, the mean resting blood pressure was 94 ± 3 mmHg.

[**Analysis**]

This is data but not result. Are the data similar or different? What is the point? The purpose of the results section is to make the point clear. To make the point clear, state the result first and then present the data, or cite a figure or a table.

[**Revision 1**]

The mean resting blood pressure was higher in the 30 tennis players than in the 20 control subjects [94 ± 3 (SD) vs. 85 ± 5 mmHg, $P < 0.02$].

[**Analysis**]

In Revision 1 the point is clear: "was higher". The sentence now states results. The data are given in parentheses after the results. (A P value for statistical significance is added to provide evidence that the difference was not likely to have occurred by chance.) However, in most cases, the data should be presented in a figure or a table rather than in the text.

In addition to simply saying "was less than", "was greater than", "decreased", or "increased", you can, when appropriate, give a general idea of the magnitude of a difference or a change by using a percentage, as in Revision 2.

[**Revision 2**]

The mean resting blood pressure was 10% higher in the 30 tennis players than in the 20 control subjects [94 ± 3 (SD) vs. 85 ± 5 mmHg, $P < 0.02$].

[**Analysis**]

In Revision 2, this statement of the result ("was 10% higher") gives a simpler and therefore clearer idea of the magnitude of the difference than do the data alone (94 ± 3 vs. 85 ± 5 mmHg).

9.5.3 Writing the results section

Remember that the results section has both text and illustrative materials (tables and figures). Use the text component to guide the readers through your key results, i. e., those results which answer the question(s) you investigated. Each table and figure must be referenced in the text portion of the results, and you must tell the readers what the key result is that each table or figure conveys.

Before sitting down to write the first draft, it is important to plan which results are important in answering the question and which can be left out. After deciding which results to present, attention should be turned to determining whether data are best presented within the text or as tables or figures. Tables and figures (photographs, drawings, graphs, flow diagrams) are often used to present details whereas the narrative section of the results tends to be used to present the general findings. Clear tables and figures provide a very powerful visual means of presenting data and should be used to complement the text, but at the same time they must stand alone. Except on rare occasions when emphasis is required, data that are given in a table or a figure must not be repeated within the text.

Tables and figures must be mentioned within the text and should be placed after the related text. Photographs of subjects are often placed within the methods section and should be used only if written, informed consent was obtained prior to the taking of the photograph. To preserve anonymity, facial features should be covered. If a manuscript includes a table or a figure that has already been published, permission must be obtained from the copyright holder (usually the publisher) and the source acknowledged.

The results must not include a discussion of the findings, methods of data analysis and citations of references, except on rare occasions when a comparison is made of the raw data with the findings of a published study. This applies only when this comparison would not fit well within the discussion.

9.5.4　Results and legends

[**Sample 6**]

A summary of renal function data is presented in Fig. 2. Continuous positive airway pressure (7.5 cm H_2O) in newborn goats decreased urine flow, sodium excretion, and the glomerular filtration rate.

[**Analysis**]

The first sentence is essentially a figure legend: Fig. 2. Renal function data. For a more powerful topic sentence, omit the figure legend and state the results. Cite the figure in parentheses at the end of the sentence that states the results.

[**Revision**]

Continuous positive airway pressure (7.5 cm H_2O) in newborn goats decreased urine flow, sodium excretion, and the glomerular filtration rate (Fig. 2).

[**Analysis**]

The reason that a result is a more powerful topic sentence than a figure legend or a table title is that a result states a message. In the example, the first sentence indicates only the topic of the paragraph—renal function data. The second sentence states a message—that renal variables decreased, which is what the readers wants to know. Therefore, this sentence should be placed first, in a powerful position, where the readers will find it readily. It should not be buried in the middle of the paragraph.

Furthermore, to use an entire sentence to direct the readers to the figure is wasteful. All that is necessary is to cite the figure in parentheses at the end of the sentence that states the results, as in the revision.

9.5.5   Comparison of results

[**Sample 7**]

Comparison with itself

- These data suggest that the HEV could be more widespread than previously thought.
- The effect of H/RZ on tuberculosis diminished over time.
- The polyclonal antibody specific to ΔrHO-1 titer was up to 1.3×10^7.

Inter-group comparison

No significant difference in results

- Patients with Karnof sky scores greater than 50 did not perform differently than controls.
- The level of chimerism did not differ between patients and controls either in blood or in liver.
- Further gender analysis revealed that RL/G of γ-H2AX of the females was 1.25 ± 0.17, and that of the males was 1.27 ± 0.16. No significant difference was observed between the males and the females.

With difference in results

- However, much shorter half-lives were found in other ruminant species, namely 11.3h in cows, 4.72h in sheep, 4.7h and 2.77h in goats.
- The percentage of irradiated lymphocytes (γ-H2AX strong positive population) was 25.57%, 25.18%, 25.44%, 24.46%, and 28.52% respectively.
- In all, 86.5 % of these polyps were precisely diagnosed by EUS, whereas only 51.7% were diagnosed by US.

Trend shown by the difference in results

- Whole-body MR imaging has a higher sensitivity than skeletal scintigraphy for the detection of bone marrow metastases.

- Females who became overweight or obese between 6 and 11 yr of age were 7 times more likely to develop new asthma symptoms at age 11 or 13.
- Maximum mean relative enhancement ratio and mean slope of relative enhancement of lung cancer patients were significantly decreased compared with those of the healthy volunteers.
- The levels of lymph TNF and IL-6 of Group A were increased than those of Group B.

Chapter Review

The results section is often considered the most important part of a research paper, which means this section attracts the most attention of editors and readers. In this chapter, we've discussed the functions and organization of results, items included in the results, and the appropriate tenses and voices to be used. Though much information could be put into this section, we recommend that it be made as concise and uncluttered as possible so that readers can find the most important and valuable information about the research.

Assignments

Task 1 *Scan the following results section extracted from an SCI paper quickly to get a general impression to find out the devices the author used to present results. What's the function of data and the figures? What do you think of its writing style? And what tense and voice are used in this section?*

Baseline characteristics are shown in Table 1. The vast majority in both groups were men of good global left ventricular systolic function (LVEF 50%). Body mass index values in both groups were similar. About 30% of study subjects had diabetes, while more than 80% had hypertension. A mean SYNTAX score was 23.0 in the CABG group and 23.5 in the HCR group ($P = 0.76$). Clinical events which occurred during hospital stay and follow-up are presented in Table 2. No patients died during in-hospital stay. There were no significant differences in in-hospital outcomes and during follow-up. The length of hospitalization was similar in both groups: 7.0 days (7.0—9.0) vs. 7.0 days (6.0—9.0), $P = 0.17$. For both treatment groups, assessment at 1 year revealed an improvement in QoL compared with the intervention assessment in all 8 domains (Fig. 2). There was a substantial difference in HRQoL between treatment groups on admission. The general QoL of patients randomized to HCR was significantly higher at baseline and in 12 month follow-up than in patients randomized to CABG (59.2 vs.51.3; $P<0.005$) and (73.7 vs. 65.6; $P<0.005$). Both groups had the same QoL improvement: in HCR group 13.5 (3.82—22.34) vs. CABG group 10.48 (2.46—31.07); $P = 0.76$. Independent predictors of improvement in 6 out of 8 domains are presented in Figure 3(略). There were no independent predictors of improvement in domain RE, VT and PCS. Observation revealed that obesity worsened QoL in PF and MCS domain, female gender improved QoL in BP domain. In addition, analysis shows whether the degree of education (lower vs. higher), marital status (relationship vs. alone) employment (employed vs. unemployed) and place of living (city vs. village) had an influence on improvement in quality of life in both groups (HCR and CABG). Depending on these factors, patients in both groups did not differ significantly (Table 3). Over 80% of all patients regardless of these factors felt improvement in HRQoL after the procedure.

Table 1. Baseline clinical characteristics

	CABG	HCR	P
Age at randomization [years]	63.5(59.0~71.0)	64.0(57.0~69.0)	0.43
Male	66(78.6%)	58(77.3%)	0.85
Body mass index [kg/m²]	28.9±4.02	28.01±3.23	0.13
Hypertension	68(81%)	67(89.3%)	0.14
Diabetes	25(29.8%)	20(26.7%)	0.67
Dyslipiemia	49(58.3%)	41(54.7%)	0.64
Obesity	37(44%)	26(34.7%)	0.23
Current smoker	32(38.1%)	23(30.7%)	0.33
Atrial fibrillation	5(6%)	4(5.3%)	0.87
Ejection fraction [%]	50(45~55)	50(48~54)	0.66
Previous MI	49(58.3%)	37(49.3%)	0.26
Previous PCI	35(41.7%)	29(38.7%)	0.7
Previous stroke	4(4.8%)	3(4%)	0.82
Previous TIA	2(2.4%)	0	0.18
Carotid artery disease	10(11.9%)	8(10.7%)	0.81
Stable angina	69(82.1%)	63(84%)	0.76
Unstable angina	15(17.9%)	12(16%)	0.76
Logistic Euro Score [points]	3(2~5)	3(1~5)	0.15
SYNTAX score	23.0(19.3~26.0)	23.5(18.0~26.5)	0.76
2 vessel CAD	45(53.6%)	35(46.7%)	0.39
3 vessel CAD	39(46.4%)	40(53.3%)	

Categorical variables were expressed as frequencies (percentages), continuous variables were expressed as mean ± standard deviation for normally distributed data and median (1ˢᵗ and 3ʳᵈ quartile) for non-normally distributed data. CABG—coronary artery bypass grafting; CAD—coronary artery disease; HCR—hybrid coronary revascularization; LIMA—left internal mammary artery; MI—myocardial infarction; MIDCAB—minimally invasive coronary artery bypass; PCI—percutaneous coronary intervention; TIA—transient ischemic attack

Table 2. Clinical endpoints occurring in the hospital or after discharge

	CABG	HCR	P
In-hospital outcomes			
Stroke	0(0%)	0(0%)	1
Perioperative MI	4(4.8%)	3(4%)	0.87
Major bleeding	3(3.6%)	1(1.3%)	0.62
Renal failure	0(0%)	0(0%)	1
Blood transfusion	20(24%)	11(15%)	0.15
Death	0(0%)	0(0%)	1
12 month follow up outcomes			
Stroke	0	0	1
MI	0	1(1.3%)	0.47
TVR	0	2(2.7%)	0.22
Repeat hospitalization	5(6%)	6(8%)	0.76

CABG—coronary artery bypass grafting; HCR—hybrid coronary revascularization; MI—myocardial infarction; TVR—target vessel revascularization

Table 3. Health-related quality of life improvement rates in various populations

	CABG	HCR	P
Degree of education			
Lower education	83.7%	90.6%	0.38
Higher education	83.3%	85.7%	0.79
Marital status			
Relationship	82%	88.7%	0.32
Alone	91%	85%	0.64
Employment			
Employed	83.3%	80%	0.82
Unemployed	83.3%	90.4%	0.27
Place of living			
City	83.1%	86.7%	0.61
Rural	85.7%	91%	0.63

CABG—coronary artery bypass grafting; HCR—hybrid coronary revascularization

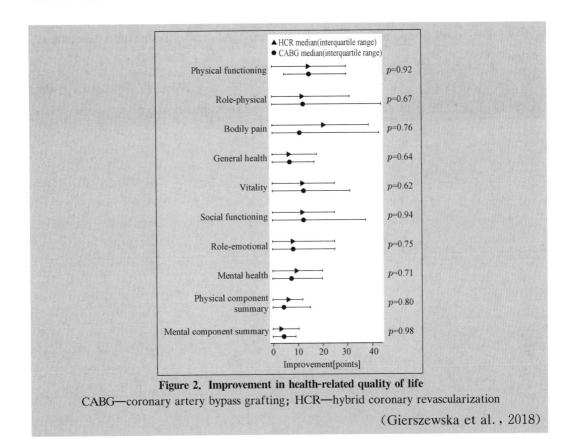

Figure 2. Improvement in health-related quality of life

CABG—coronary artery bypass grafting; HCR—hybrid coronary revascularization

（Gierszewska et al. , 2018）

Task 2 *Select one or two English academic papers in your academic area, read the results section through to see if you have successfully understood the writing of results. If you can, try to summarize the writing rules, and then try to rewrite or modify a result according to the data and figure of the paper you selected.*

Task 3 *Complete the following sentences by translating the expression in parentheses into English.*

1. The _____（显著增长）of these diseases illustrates the vast collateral damage to health caused by policies made in other sectors and in the international systems.

2. _____（入院 2 周后），the patient's left leg pain had completely resolved，and the swelling went down gradually.

3. There are _____（均无显著差异）in the average operation time，bleeding in operation and the preserved time of installing catheter after operation between the two groups.

4. The result of counting show that counting value is consistent with experiment value, _____（平均误差仅 0.2%）.

5. There is _____（呈负相关）between the severity of neurological deficit and blood glucose concentration.

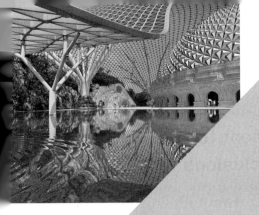

Chapter Ten

Discussion and Conclusions Writing

Lead-in Questions

1. Do you know the difference between results and conclusions?

2. Do you know anything about the writing requirements of the discussion and conclusions?

Learning Objectives

After learning this unit, you will be able to:

1. distinguish the several forms of processing the discussion and conclusions,

2. and develop the section of discussion and conclusions in a proper way.

✓参考答案
✓课件申请
✓学术资源

10.1 Structural arrangement for the discussion and conclusions

Discussion and conclusions sections are the fourth subheading and the highlight of the whole research paper, which are related to whether the article could have a happy ending. Discussion section intends to explain results convincingly, while, in many cases, conclusions are taken as a summary of the results and discussion. Thus, results, discussion and conclusions are not only related in content, but also in structure. Conventionally, results, discussion and conclusions are three separate parts. Sometimes, the discussion is concluded in results, namely, providing all the results together with discussion. And sometimes, conclusions are included in discussion, providing the conclusions together with discussion. At another time, both results and discussion are separate parts, with conclusions included in either of them or not. It is also common to see that there are two separate parts—results and conclusions, in which the discussion is included in results.

The following table shows different structural arrangement for the results, discussion and conclusions sections in different SCI papers.

Table 10‑1 Structural arrangement patterns in SCI papers

	Subheading	Form
A	• Results • Discussion • Conclusions	Three separate sections
B	• Results (and Discussion)	Combined (Discussion is included in Results)
C	• Discussion (and Conclusions)	Combined (Conclusions section is included in Discussion).
D	• Results • Discussion	Two separate sections (Conclusions section is included or not).
E	• Results • Conclusions	Two separate sections (Discussion is included).

Sometimes it is difficult for the researcher to present enough findings to support her/his research hypothesis completely, and the research could benefit from further study. In such a circumstance, the discussion section and conclusions section can be merged into a single section.

In many research fields, the two sections—discussion section and conclusions section, are not separated, and the difference is partly conventional, depending on traditions of particular fields and journals.

10.2   The format and function of the conclusions

As for the conclusions section, there are several common views; accordingly, there are several forms of processing (included in the discussion section, stated as a separate subheading):

- For many papers, conclusions are taken as a summary of the results and discussion sections, so sometimes it can be included in the discussion;
- Conclusions could take the implications, significance or consequence of the study into consideration;
- Conclusions usually suggest a speculation of future trends and need for future research.

[**Sample 1—Conclusions**]

(1) We have integrated preclinical gnotobiotic animal models with human studies to understand the contributions of perturbed gut microbiota development to childhood undernutrition and to identify new microbiota-directed therapeutic approaches. (2) We identified a set of proteins that distinguish the plasma proteomes of healthy children from those with SAM. (3) Using these data, we have developed a supplemental food prototype, MDCF-2, that shifted the plasma proteome of children with MAM toward that of healthy individuals, including proteins involved in linear growth, bone development, neurodevelopment, and immune function. MDCF-2 is a tool for investigating, in larger studies across different populations with varying degrees of undernutrition, how repair of gut microbiota immaturity affects various facets of child growth. (Gehrig et al. , 2019)

[**Analysis**]

The sample above briefly summarizes several important elements. The first sentence generalizes the study method, study purpose and key results. The second sentence restates the findings and the finding's function or applications. The third sentence is the contribution of the findings. So, this sample is a more comprehensive one. The formal content of the above three conclusions is all covered.

Here, it is a good idea for you to read and understand the discussion/conclusions section with reference to the introduction. Usually, it is the most direct way to re-examine and understand the previous content, especially the introduction section.

10.3 The function, role and principle of the discussion

10.3.1 The function of the discussion

Discussion is an important section of an academic paper, which is generally considered the most difficult to write. It is the refinement of research significance and value based on the review of research process and results. If the quality of the abstract could determine whether the readers choose to read or not, the success or failure of the discussion determines whether the editor or reviewer of the SCI journal agrees to publish the paper or not. From the discussion section, readers can also get a rational understanding of the significance of the study.

Discussion is closely connected with results because the results of a research should be explained, supported, compared and evaluated in this section. Therefore, the discussion section should provide both empirical and logic evidence to support the explanation, evaluation or answer of the study and indicate the application prospect and potential significance or limitation of the research.

Therefore, the function of the discussion section is to explain the phenomenon, illustrate the point, explain the implications of your survey/research findings, and make recommendations for future research.

10.3.2 The role and principle of the discussion

Discussion is generally regarded as the "heart" of a paper, which can best reflect the author's mastery of literature and understanding of the progress of a certain academic issue. The purpose of the discussion section of academic papers is to reveal the significance of research findings and respond to existing research topics. Its primary role and writing principles are generally as follows:

- to answer questions posed in the introduction;
- to explain how the research supports the answers;
- to explain how the results are consistent or inconsistent with published studies;
- to clearly state the conclusions and generalizations derived from the research results.

In particular, writing in the discussion section usually includes the above principles. But for the latter two, writing is not necessarily exhaustive or comprehensive, especially for pioneering research.

In terms of structure, discussion often follows the "findings" (results or findings) and echoes the "introduction" of the paper. The discussion section is responsible for explaining "what it means/so what". Therefore, a common sentence pattern in the discussion section is: "...[the results] suggests that ...[conclusions]".

10.4   The organization of the discussion and conclusions

Based on the above discussion and its corresponding textual features, the discussion section can be composed of three parts:
- restating and explaining the questions involved and results (such as hypothesis and main findings);
- describing the relevance and importance of the findings, and comparing the findings with those from previous researches;
- indicating the research limitation and direction of future research.

The basic structure of the discussion and conclusions follows a specific-to-general pattern with 6 moves included:
- Move 1: Reviewing background;
- Move 2: Summarizing and generalizing the key findings/results;
- Move 3: Analyzing and interpreting key findings/results and comparing them with related researches;
- Move 4: Stating the conclusions of the study;
- Move 5: Stating limitations of the study;
- Move 6: Suggesting a speculation of future trends and need for future research.

In addition, the success of the discussion and conclusions is closely related to the ingenious application of the various rhetoric means to make the moves coherent, logical and scientific. Both certainty words and tentative words play an important role in academic English writing. It is not always necessary to use adjectives or adverbs such as "sure" and "certainly" to express certainty. Instead, the present, past and perfect tenses of most main verbs (know, believe, give, etc.) indicate the meaning and show certainty. In research papers, tentative words are used to express the results not directly obtained from the experiments. Modal auxiliaries can be used to show uncertainty/tentative meaning with different degrees. Those words according to degree for certainty from low to high are might, may, could, can, should, ought to, would, will and must (Wu, 2013). Some commonly used sentence patterns of modal auxiliaries are very helpful for learners to express or identify information when writing or reading a paper.

1) Subject + (modal auxiliary) be done + that + Noun clause (information element)

E. g.   Although more research is needed to show the impact stress can have on female fertility, researchers recommend minimizing stress and practicing healthy coping methods when trying to conceive.

2) It + (modal auxiliary) be + that + Noun clause (information element)

E. g.　It could be suggested that syncopic reaction could be reduced by improving the working condition for blood donation to prevent mental stress, avoiding empty stomach, fatigue, etc.

3) It + (modal auxiliary) be + adj + that + Noun clause (information element)

E. g.　It would be beneficial for patients to extend treatment when the dosage of antibiotics is reduced.

10.5　Textual structure elements and functional discourse coherence

10.5.1　References between textual structural elements

The discussion often follows the "findings"(results) and echoes the "introduction" of the paper, as mentioned above.

In the writing process, the content and structure of the discussion and conclusions on the macro level (such as function, specific format, writing moves and principles, etc.) should be clarified first, and then the content to be expressed on the micro level should be accurately and objectively expressed. Only on this basis can the writing quality be effectively guaranteed.

In order to facilitate learners to better understand and grasp the writing skills of the discussion/conclusions section, the following sample is extracted from *Science*, especially with its introduction, results and discussion included. While reading, pay attention to moves of important elements and ignore some of the difficult or specialized words. When the introduction and results are considered as reference, the moves in discussion could be understood even more comprehensively. Pay special attention to the first or first two sentences while reading (Miyahara et al., 2017).

[Sample 2—Discussion/Conclusions]

Discussion

In the present study, 35% of the children were hospitalized at least once during their first 2 years of life, and 80% of the hospitalizations were caused by common infectious diseases such as LRTIs, GIs and non-focal viral infections. ETS exposure due to $PS_{p/i}$ was associated with significantly increased risks of infectious disease-related hospitalization and, more specifically, LRTI-related hospitalization. However, the influence of $PS_{p/i}$ on the risk of other infectious and non-infectious diseases was not demonstrated in the same population.

We found that $PS_{p/i}$ independently increased the risk of LRTI-related hospitalization in this prospective cohort study after controlling for low socio-economic status, young maternal age, low weight gain during pregnancy and LBW, although these confounders might increase the rate of hospitalization. This finding is consistent with the results of our previous cross-sectional study, which showed that exposure to in-house tobacco smoking in the same province increased the prevalence of pneumonia in children under 5 years of age (adjusted OR = 1.55, 95% CI: 1.25 - 1.92). These results are also consistent with the findings of a study performed in Hong Kong that assessed the association of ETS exposure with respiratory tract or febrile illness (OR 1.28, 95% CI: 1.01 - 1.61); most of the smoking exposure in that setting was also due to fathers and other household members.

Maternal smoking exposure in utero and during postnatal periods has been shown to present a risk of childhood diseases; maternal smoking during pregnancy has been associated with a decrease in lung function and an increased incidence of wheezing and asthma. Although $PS_{p/i}$ was not found to influence respiratory symptoms, acute respiratory infections or respiratory function among young children in some studies, the importance of $PS_{p/i}$ has been shown in other studies. A large Norwegian cohort study suggested that paternal smoking was significantly associated with a risk of LRTIs among children 6—18 months of age after adjusting for maternal smoking, although the effects were smaller than those of maternal smoking during pregnancy. In the present study, we were able to directly evaluate the effect of $PS_{p/i}$ without adjusting for the effect of maternal smoking exposure.

In the Norwegian study mentioned above, both prenatal maternal smoking exposure and postnatal paternal smoking exposure without maternal smoking increased the risk of LRTIs, but prenatal paternal exposure in utero did not. Fuentes-Leonarte et al. reported that postnatal exposure from fathers was related to otitis. In our study, paternal smoking status was determined at enrollment and we did not distinguish the effects of ETS exposure during pregnancy from those in infancy, because we assumed that smoking habits would not change after a child's birth or during childhood. Given the similar rates of smoking status between 2006 and 2010 found in census data, misclassification of paternal smoking exposure after birth would not be frequent. The effect of second-hand smoking during pregnancy and infancy could be clarified by measuring the urinary cotinine levels of mothers and children, as these measurements would provide more objective data on ETS exposure status.

Previous studies have shown that maternal smoking during pregnancy is a risk factor for LBW and that paternal smoking has a smaller effect on LBW. In the present study, we also found that there were more LBW children among those exposed to paternal smoking than in those without exposure (2.6% vs. 1.9%), although this difference did not reach significance ($P = 0.345$).

The high burden of hospital admissions due to respiratory infections (LRTIs + URTIs,

110.9 per 1000 PYO) among children under 2 years of age in Vietnam was similar to the burden of acute respiratory infections identified among children under 1 year old in a previous study conducted in both an urban area, Ho Chi Minh City (81 per 1000 PYO), and a rural area, Dong Thap (138 per 1000 PYO). Preventive measures against second-hand smoking during pregnancy and infancy are expected to have a high impact nationwide, not only in Nha Trang, because of the high incidence rate of respiratory infections throughout Vietnam.

Our study has several limitations. First, we captured only hospitalized cases so that the results might be hampered by the selection bias: factors influencing on their medical care-seeking behaviours might be associated with the number of patients with serious illness who did not consult a doctor at the hospital. It would not be true because children can receive free medical treatments at public hospitals like KHGH. This notion was supported by our previous cross sectional surveillance in the province. Second, the impact of paternal smoking exposure might be underestimated in the present study because the children who were lost to follow-up and the $PS_{p/i}$-exposed children shared similar characteristics, such as low socio-economic status, young maternal age and living with siblings. However, the percentage of children exposed to $PS_{p/i}$ did not differ between those followed and those lost to follow-up (60.8% vs. 57.3%, $P = 0.211$), mitigating the risk of this limitation. Another possible source of underestimation of impact of paternal smoking comes from an absence of information on the exposure to tobacco smoking of other members of household without $PS_{p/i}$. However, as we previously reported, parental smoking accounted for a large portion (73.5%) of tobacco smoke in households among the children aged < 5 years lived in the province in 2006. Third, there are additional potential confounding factors that we did not address in this study such as crowding and sanitation. The major strength of this study was its prospective study design and relatively high follow-up rate, which minimized the selection and recall biases inherent to retrospective studies. As Khanh Hoa General Hospital (KHGH) is the only tertiary health facility available to the study population, and as the study population has good access to primary and secondary health facilities for referral, we were able to capture almost all severe illness events.

$PS_{p/i}$ contributed to the incidence of severe LRTIs requiring hospitalization in children less than 2 years old in Nha Trang, Vietnam, and was responsible for 24% of the total LRTI incidence; in contrast, LBW was responsible for only 1.3% of all LRTI cases. As LRTIs are the most common cause of hospitalization and are associated with longer hospital stays, smoking reduction interventions targeted at households with pregnant women and children may effectively improve child health.

[**Analysis**]

In Sample 2 above, supported by the results, the discussion section shows a specific-to-general pattern by following the important moves, with the important composing elements/

parts of the discussion included. It also echoes the introduction of the paper. All these could be easily identified with the help of using functional morphology and syntax. We can clearly follow the important moves and identify the important composing elements/parts from the following sentence structures selected from the first sentence of each paragraphs.

1) In the present study, 35% of the children were ... ,

2) We found that ... ,

3) ... has been shown to present a risk of ... ,

4) In the Norwegian study mentioned above, both ... and ... increased the risk of ... , but prenatal paternal exposure in utero did not.

5) The ... was similar to ... ,

6) Our study has several limitations. First, ...

7) ... may effectively improve child health.

The following attached introduction and result sections (Sample 3) are from the same paper of Sample 2. Read the following introduction and results sections with the help of the analysis above, and try to achieve a deeper understanding of discussion/conclusions.

[**Sample 3**]

Introduction

Infectious diseases such as pneumonia and diarrhoea are major contributors to child morbidity and mortality in low- and middle-income countries, with most cases occurring in the first 2 years of life. These diseases are associated with a high economic burden. In Southeast Asia, after excluding neonatal deaths, pneumonia and diarrhoea account for half of all deaths in children under 5 years of age 5.

Environmental tobacco smoke (ETS) exposure is an important and early modifiable risk factor for childhood illnesses such as respiratory symptoms, respiratory infections, asthma and sudden infant death. The biological mechanisms of the disease risk conferred by ETS exposure have been investigated by *in vitro* functional studies on Toll-like receptors and blood cell, and these studies have suggested that tobacco smoke alters local and systemic innate immunity. Therefore, the effect of ETS exposure may not be limited to respiratory diseases. However, there is limited and conflicting evidence regarding the association of ETS exposure with the risks of other types of infectious diseases such as acute otitis media and gastroenteritis. Furthermore, few prospective studies of child populations have assessed the risks associated with ETS exposure in populations in which the contribution of female or maternal smoking exposure is negligible like Vietnamese. We previously reported that ETS exposure due to household members was significantly associated with an increased risk of parent-reported child pneumonia (OR = 1.55, 95% CI: 1.25 – 1.92) in a cross-sectional population surveillance study in Vietnam; however, the detection of cases was not fully reliable because it was based on parental self-report questionnaires. As tobacco smoking is highly prevalent among young Vietnamese men and as only 1.0% of smokers in Nha Trang, Vietnam, are women 18 – 50 years of age, parental smoking, particularly paternal smoking, could be a risk factor for childhood diseases including, but not limited to, respiratory infections.

In the present study, we described the burden and pattern of severe illness including infectious and non-infectious diseases that require hospitalization using the medical records of Vietnamese children registered in a prospective birth cohort study. Additionally, we aimed to improve the strength of evidence for the association of parental smoking with the incidence of childhood health problems.

Results

Baseline characteristics of the Nha Trang birth cohort. We enrolled 1999 children at birth; 1624 of those children (81.2%) were confirmed to have been residing in the study catchment area for 24 months or from birth to death. The remaining 375 children were excluded from the analysis: 5 died, with uncertain information about the date of death, the cause of death or both; 251 had left the study catchment area; and 119 could not be traced. Children who attended follow-up visits had a significantly higher household economic status, higher mother's education level, older maternal age and a higher likelihood of living with siblings than children who did not. The prevalence of exposure to paternal tobacco smoking during pregnancy and infancy ($PS_{p/i}$) was 57.3%. None of the women reported smoking tobacco during pregnancy, and ETS exposure was not caused by maternal smoking in this population. Exposure to $PS_{p/i}$ was associated with young maternal age, low household income, low maternal education level, living with siblings and low weight gain during pregnancy.

Incidence of hospitalizations. A total of 939 hospitalization events were recorded during the 24-month observation period. The most common cause of these hospitalizations was lower respiratory tract infections (LRTIs) (11.1% of the study participants), accounting for 24.7% of all hospitalizations. Gastrointestinal infections (GIs) and non-focal viral infections were the second and third most common causes of hospitalization, accounting for 20.8% and 17.4% of all hospitalizations, respectively. The median length of hospital stay for LRTIs was 4 days, which was longer than that of other infectious diseases (3 days, $P < 0.001$ by Kruskal-Wallis test) including GIs (LRTIs vs GIs, Wilcoxon rank sum test $P < 0.001$) and upper respiratory tract infections (URTIs) (LRTIs vs URTIs, Wilcoxon rank sum test $P < 0.001$).

Risk factor analysis of cause-specific hospitalizations. The results of univariable analyses for cause-specific hospitalization are shown in Supplementary Tables S2 and S3. $PS_{p/i}$ was identified as a risk factor for LRTIs but not for other causes of hospitalization, whereas age at hospitalization, calendar month at hospitalization, living with a sibling, maternal age at delivery and maternal body mass index were associated with other types of infectious and non-infectious diseases but not with LRTIs. In the multivariable analyses, exposure to $PS_{p/i}$ independently increased the risk of total infectious disease-related hospitalizations 1.26-fold ($P = 0.012$); $PS_{p/i}$ increased the risk of LRTIs 1.76 – fold (95% C.I. 1.24 – 2.51; $P = 0.002$), whereas the incidence of other infectious diseases including URTIs as well as non-infectious diseases was not associated with $PS_{p/i}$. LRTIs represented the increase in infectious disease risk due to $PS_{p/i}$. Although maternal age at delivery, low birth weight (LBW, less than 2.5 kg) and monthly household income were possible risk factors for LRTIs in the univariable analysis ($P < 0.1$), the effect size of $PS_{p/i}$ on LRTIs did not change after adjusting for these potential confounders, confirming that the effect of $PS_{p/i}$ was independent of LBW and other residual confounders. The population attributable fraction (PAF) of all infections associated with $PS_{p/i}$ was 11.8%, and the PAF of LRTIs associated with $PS_{p/i}$ was 14.7%. $PS_{p/i}$ exposure increased the population attributable risks (PARs) of all infections and of LRTIs by 48.9 per 1000 person-years of observation (PYO) and 39.4 per 1000 PYO, respectively. Although LBW was a strong risk factor for LRTI-related hospitalizations, increasing the risk 2.27-fold ($P = 0.062$), LBW increased the PAF of LRTIs by 1.3%. Thus, LBW had a smaller impact on LRTI incidence than $PS_{p/i}$. A Kaplan-Meier plot depicted the hospitalization events related to LRTI that occurred in the early months of $PS_{p/i}$—exposed children's lives, and the effect of $PS_{p/i}$ persisted during the entire observation period.

10.5.2　Functional discourse coherence

In discourse construction, cohesive relation is the basic necessity in forming a coherent passage. Conjunctive words play an important part in the realization of discourse coherence. They imply some kinds of discourse coherence, such as emphasis, contrast, comparison, concession, logic order, cause and consequence. Using conjunctive words to establish a coherent discourse is a basic criterion to assess a learner's ability to write EAP. The following logical conjunctive words are often involved in the discussion and conclusions section.

Table 10 – 2　Logical conjunctive words in the discussion and conclusion section

Logic relationship	Conjunctive words
Order	afterward ... at first, eventually, finally, first of all, first, followed by, immediately, in the end, in the middle of, next to, next, opposite to, second, soon, then, to begin with
Concession	after all, although, if not, it is true (that)...
Time	after, as, before, it is since ... , not ... until ... , since, until, when, while

(Continued)

Logic relationship	conjunctive words
Cause	as，because of this，because，due to，for this reason …，for，owing to，since
Consequence	accordingly，as a result，consequently，hence，in this way，so，therefore，thus
Emphasis	above all，anyway，as a matter of fact，certainly，especially，in fact，in particular，in this case …，indeed，naturally，obviously，of course，particularly，surely
Example	a case in point，as an illustration，for example，for instance，for one thing，including，like，namely，particularly …，that is，to illustrate
Comparison	at the same time，even though，in the same way，likewise …，meanwhile，not only … but also，similarly
Contrast	although，but，conversely，despite，however，if not …，in contrast，in spite of，instead，nevertheless，on the contrary，on the other hand，opposite to，or else，otherwise，still，whereas，while，yet

Semantic cohesion is one of the most important cohesive devices in English discourse. And it plays a fundamental and critical role in constructing a coherent text.

Besides conjunctive words that could be used symbolically，semantic relevance is another important means to achieve discourse coherence. It is the intrinsic feature of discourse coherence. In case of discussion/conclusions，its semantic relevance could be achieved based on its functions，namely，the appropriate or specific writing structure，requirements or principles of discussion/conclusions. Only in proper context can functional cohesion achieve coherence in discourse.

Table 10 - 3　Constructing a coherent text

Moves	Requirements	Examples of functional semantic cohesive phrases
Move 1	Reviewing background	There is a … to … that involves …，Current … given to … with … have not been … based on knowledge of how …，It has also been suggested …
Move 2	Summarizing and generalizing the key findings/results	A surprising finding was that …
Move 3	Analyzing and interpreting key findings/results and comparing them with related researches	Findings of … are consistent with … refer to, the findings are further supported by …，contrary to our hypothesis，…
Move 4	Stating the conclusions of the study	These results show/suggest/indicate …，In this study, we have found that/demonstrate that/ provide evidence that …，The evidence indicates that/ suggests that …，It was verified that …，These findings demonstrate …，… there was no relationship between …

(**Continued**)

Moves	Requirements	Examples of functional semantic cohesive phrases
Move 5	Stating limitations of the study	This paper acknowledges several limitations that ... ,
Move 6	Suggesting a speculation of future trends and need for future research	This highlights ... , ... demonstrates the potential to be a ... , Further researches should ... , ... described here will enable major advances in ...

In order to facilitate learners' connection with the preceding and following chapters, this chapter continues to select a sample from the *Cardiology Journal*, published in 2013. This time, the sample is the discussion section of the paper. Pay attention to its functional semantic cohesive words or phrases and conjunctive words underlined and ignore its difficult words or phrases.

[**Sample 4—Discussion**]

Discussion

In this study, we investigated the predictors of recurrence in patients undergoing cryoballon ablation for paroxysmal AF. The main findings were as follows: clinical success in regard to the freedom from recurrent AF was 80%, early recurrence of AF was the most important predictor of late recurrence of AF, intra-left AEMD, PA lateral, EHRA symptom score and age predicted late recurrence of AF. Atrial fibrillation duration prior to ablation, gender, coronary artery disease, hypertension, alcohol consumption, LA diameter, LA volume, EF, biomarkers, epicardial fat, pericardial effusion did not predict late recurrence of AF.

One year success of AF ablation in other studies was 60% ~ 70%. Eighty percent success of our study may be the result of normal LA dimensions, inclusion of only PAF patients, no structural heart disease, and single center study.

Previous studies showed that postablation inflammation around PVs caused increase in inflammatory markers and cardiac enzymes. When cryoballon ablation is performed, lesion formation occurs at the entire circumference of the balloon and that results in a long circumferential lesion. The higher rise of biomarkers indicates more myocardial injury. However, this did not translate into late ablation success in our study. These markers represent overall inflammation and injury, they don't represent each PV separately. Therefore, higher rise may represent the sum of one transmural lesion and one superficial lesion.

AF ablation creates large lesions and this may play a role in effusion formation. Ten percent of our patients had pericardial effusion. Pericardial effusion may be a sign of lesion thickness. Pericardial effusion and late recurrence of AF were not related ($p > 0.05$) in our study, it may be due to the fact that it is a nonspesific sign of injury as biomarkers.

Batal et al. demonstrated that increased posterior LA fat thickness was associated with

AF burden independent of age, body mass index, or LA area. <u>They thought that</u> local inflammatory mediators produced by the pericardial epicardial fat in the LA posterior wall promoted the activation of ectopic foci in the PV ostia. In our study <u>we could not find any relationship between</u> pericardial adiposity and late recurrence of AF.

Ethanol and its metabolite acetaldehyde <u>have been shown to</u> increase levels of circulating catecholamines. Ethanol <u>may also</u> induce oxidative stress and release of plasma free fatty acids. These indirect effects of ethanol may be arrhythmogenic, particularly in individuals prone to AF <u>such as</u> patients with focal AF. A meta-analysis <u>supported</u> these pathophysiologic expression <u>and showed that</u> habitual heavy alcohol drinking was associated with an increased risk of AF.

In our study <u>there was no relationship between</u> alcohol intake and late recurrence of AF. <u>It may be related to</u> our patient population, <u>because all of</u> our patients were moderate alcohol drinkers and nondrinkers.

In our study <u>we could not find any statistical significant relationship between</u> late recurrence of AF and LA diameter, LA volume and EF, <u>it may be related to</u> their normal values. Perhaps LA anatomical remodelling was less in our group. <u>There was no relationship with</u> AF duration <u>also</u>, <u>it may be because</u> it doesn't demonstrate the AF frequency and AF episode duration, <u>so</u> it doesn't reflect atrial remodeling.

High EHRA symptom score <u>was related</u> to late recurrence of AF, <u>perhaps it is because</u> these patients have more symptomatic PAF episodes than the others. (Evranos et al.,2013)

[**Analysis**]

Sample 3 is a combined discussion, in which conclusions are included in the discussion. The underlined words or phrases are some of the main functional semantic cohesive phrases and conjunctive words.

10.6　Things to be avoided when writing discussion

The success or failure of the discussion first determines whether the paper is accepted by a journal or not. It is the poor writing and presentation skills that lead to the rejection of a considerable number of works. Among them, the most common writing mistakes include inaccurate or incomplete comments on research significance, too much listing of experimental data, too long and cumbersome expression of results or research significance.

10.6.1　Over-interpretation of the results

It is easy to inflate the interpretation of the results. Be careful that your interpretation of the results does not go beyond what is supported by the data. The data are the data: nothing more, nothing less.

10.6.2   Unwarranted speculation

There is little room for speculation in the discussion. The discussion should remain focused on your data and the patients and/or devices in your study. If the subjects in your study had asthma, it is usually not appropriate to speculate about how your findings might apply to other patient populations. If your study used volume-controlled ventilation, it may not be appropriate to speculate about how the findings might apply to pressure-controlled ventilation. If you feel compelled to speculate, be certain that you clearly identify your comments as speculation: "We speculate that ..."

10.6.3   Inflating the importance of the findings

After all of the hard work that goes into a study, it is easy to attribute unwarranted importance to study findings. We all want our study to make an important contribution that will be cited for generations to come. However, unwarranted inflation of the importance of the study results will disgust reviewers and readers. A measure of humility goes a long way.

10.6.4   Tangential issues

It is important to remain focused on the hypothesis and study results. Injecting tangential issues into the discussion section distracts and confuses readers. Tangential issues run the risk of diluting and confounding the real message of the study.

Let's read the first part of the discussion section extracted from an article about the estimation of epidemic trend of COVID-19 in Wuhan, China under an infectious disease dynamics SEIR model. The model shows that the estimated number of infections would reach the peak in late February, and sufficient and strict measures should be taken in China.

[**Sample 5   Discussion**]

Discussion

Estimations of the transmission risk and the epidemic trend of COVID-19 are of great importance because these can arouse the vigilance of the policy makers, health professionals, and the whole society so that enough resources would be mobilized in a speedy and efficient way for both control and treatment. We estimated the number of infections using SEIR (Susceptible, Exposed, Infectious, and Removed) model under two assumptions of Rt (Rt maintaining to be >1 or Rt gradually decreasing to <1) in the purpose of depicting various possible epidemic trends of COVID-19 in Wuhan, China. Two estimations provide an approach for evaluating the sufficiency of the current measures taken in China, depending on whether or not the peak of the number of infections would occur in February 2020. Assuming the current control measures were ineffective and insufficient, the estimated number of infections would continue to increase throughout February without a peak. On the other hand, assuming the current control measures were effective and sufficient, the estimated number of infections would reach the peak in late February 2020. (Wang et al., 2020)

[Analysis]

This part is the first paragraph of the discussion. From it we may find that 1) it remains focused on the data the authors calculated in the study; 2) an objective evaluation of the findings has been made here; 3) it focuses on the study and the results from the first sentence to the end.

Chapter Review

In this chapter, we have discussed the format, function, organization and writing principles of the discussion and conclusions section in SCI papers. Some suggestions are also made to avoid the most common writing mistakes.

In many research fields, the two sections—discussion and conclusions, are not distinguished, and the difference is partly conventional, depending on traditions of particular fields and journals.

Discussion is the most important section of an academic paper. It is closely connected with result and echoes the "introduction" of the paper. This section should be written in a specific-to-general pattern with 6 moves.

- The function of the discussion section is to substantially convey what you think your results mean and why you think things worked out the way they did in your study. The discussion section is used to analyze both the result and the hypothesis, to show your attitude to present former research and propose the direction for further study.

- The function of the conclusions section is to explain whether you have solved the problem completely, or, if not completely, how much progress you have made in your field because of your work. Don't mention the process of how you have reached the conclusions, as this should be stated in the discussion section. State your conclusions as well as both the limitations of your study and your suggestions for future research.

Assignments

Task 1 *The following sentences are taken from the conclusions section of an academic paper entitled "Improved Reference Genome of Aedes Aegypti Informs Arbovirus Vector Control", published in* Nature. *Rearrange these sentences into a coherent conclusion.*（Matthews et al. , 2018）

A. "Sterile Insect Technique" and "Incompatible Insect Technique" show great promise to suppress mosquito populations, but these population suppression methods require that only males are released.

B. The high-quality genome assembly and annotation described here will enable major advances in mosquito biology, and has already allowed us to carry out a number of experiments that were previously impossible.

C. A new appreciation of copy number variation in insecticide-detoxifying GSTe genes and a more complete accounting of Cys-loop LGICs will catalyse the search for new resistance-breaking insecticides.

D. A strategy that connects a gene for male determination to a gene drive construct has been proposed to effectively bias the population towards males over multiple generations, and improved understanding of M locus evolution and the function of its genetic content should facilitate genetic control of mosquitoes that infect many hundreds of millions of people with arboviruses every year.

E. The highly contiguous AaegL5 genome permitted high-resolution genome-wide analysis of genetic variation and the mapping of loci for DENV vector competence and insecticide resistance.

F. A doubling in the known number of chemosensory ionotropic receptors provides opportunities to link odorants and tastants on human skin to mosquito attraction, a key first step in the development of novel mosquito repellents.

Analysis:_____.

Task 2 *Each of the following passages is the first two or three sentences extracted from every paragraph in the discussion of an SCI paper. Try to arrange these paragraphs in a typical order（the first two paragraphs have been given to you）.（The GBD 2015 Obesity Collaborators, 2017）*

1-A. In our systematic evaluation of the health effects of high BMI, we found that excess body weight accounted for about 4 million deaths and 120 million disability-adjusted life-years worldwide in 2015. Nearly 70% of the deaths that were related to high BMI were due to cardiovascular disease, and more than 60% of those deaths occurred among obese persons.

2-J. Among the leading health risks that were assessed in the Global Burden of Disease 2015 study, high BMI continues to have one of the highest rates of increase. Across levels of development, the prevalence of obesity has increased over recent decades, which indicates that the problem is not simply a function of income or wealth.

G. Our study has several important strengths. We have addressed the major limitations of previous studies by including more data sources and quantifying the prevalence of obesity among children. We also systematically evaluated the strength of evidence for the causal relationship between high BMI and health outcomes and included all BMI-outcome pairs for which sufficient evidence with respect to causal relationship was available.

E. Our study showed a greater increase in the rate of exposure to high BMI than in the rate of the related disease burden. This difference was driven mainly by the decline in risk-deleted mortality, particularly for cardiovascular disease; factors such as improved treatment or changes in other risks have resulted in decreases in the rate of cardiovascular disease despite increases in BMI.

C. The potential limitations of our study should also be considered. We used both self-reported and measured data with respect to height and weight and corrected the bias in self-reported data using measured data at each age, sex, and geographic region.

B. We found that 5% of the disability-adjusted life-years that were related to high BMI were from musculoskeletal disorders. Although high BMI is a major risk factor contributing to years lived with disability globally, and the economic costs associated with treatment are substantial, these nonfatal but debilitating health outcomes have received comparatively little policy attention.

D. Our systematic evaluation of prospective observational studies showed sufficient evidence supporting a causal relationship between high BMI and cancers of the esophagus, colon and rectum, liver, gallbladder and biliary tract, pancreas, breast, uterus, ovary, kidney, and thyroid, along with leukemia. A recent review by the International Agency for Research on Cancer (IARC) comes to largely similar conclusions, except with respect to leukemia.

F. In conclusion, our study provides a comprehensive assessment of the trends in high BMI and the associated disease burden. Our results show that both the prevalence and disease burden of high BMI are increasing globally. These findings highlight the need for implementation of multicomponent interventions to reduce the prevalence and disease burden of high BMI.

I. During the past decade, researchers have proposed a range of interventions to reduce obesity. Among such interventions are restricting the advertisement of unhealthy foods to children, improving school meals, using taxation to reduce consumption of unhealthy foods and providing subsidies to increase intake of healthy foods, and using supply-chain incentives to increase the production of healthy foods.

H. Globally, 39% of deaths and 37% of disability-adjusted life-years that were related to high BMI occurred among nonobese persons. Although some studies have suggested that overweight is associated with a lower risk of death from any cause than is a normal range of BMI (18 to 25), recent evidence from a meta-analysis and pooled analysis of prospective observational studies showed a continuous increase in the risk of death associated with a BMI of more than 25.

Analysis: _____ .

Task 3   *Read an SCI paper relevant to your major or of interest from Appendix Ⅱ, paying attention to its functional semantic cohesive words or phrases and ignoring its difficult words or phrases. Discuss with your partners, and fill them in the following table.*

Moves	Requirements	Functional semantic cohesive words or phrases
Move 1	Reviewing background	
Move 2	Summarizing and generalizing the key findings/results	
Move 3	Analyzing and interpreting key findings/results and comparing them with related researches	
Move 4	Stating the conclusions of the study	
Move 5	Stating limitations of the study	
Move 6	Suggesting a speculation of future trends and need for future research	

Task 4 *Complete the following sentences by translating the expression in parentheses into English.*

1. The evidence of a link remains elusive and _____ _____(需要更多的研究进一步探索出)the possible risk.

2. _____(还有一种观点认为) that autism(孤独) could be one possible cause of traditionally "female" problems such as anorexia.

3. _____(对于这种假设的进一步证据) has been obtained by examining the position of the median in the boxplot.

4. _____(主要研究结果如下)：clinical success in regard to the freedom from recurrent AF was 80%，early recurrence of AF was the most important predictor of late recurrence of AF, intra-left AEMD, PA lateral, EHRA symptom score and age predicted late recurrence of AF.

5. _____(根据现有的研究和建议), the target uric acid concentration of < 5 mg/dL should be considered in patients with high cardiovascular risk.

6. Yet，what was surprising was _____(接受调查的 医生对……之间的关系缺乏认识), of the relationship between hyperuricaemia and ischemic heart disease，and thus a growing cardiovascular risk.

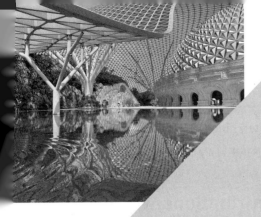

Chapter Eleven

Contributions, Acknowledgements and References in English Medical Academic Papers

✓参考答案
✓课件申请
✓学术资源

Contributions，acknowledgements and the references are the end matter after the text-body of the SCI paper，echoing to the front matter (including the title，author information and abstract) and the text. They are an essential part of SCI papers.

11.1　Acknowledgements and contributions writing

Acknowledgments and contributions are usually placed after the text-body. Acknowledgements express thanks to the institutes or individuals who have helped the author(s) in the process of research or during the writing of the paper，which reflects the author's gratitude and recognition for the help he/she received from others. Contributions describe the authors' different involvement to the published work. Appropriate and standard acknowledgements and contributions will reflect the author's good scientific spirit and accomplishment.

Acknowledgements and contributions are presented separately in some SCI journals，while some contributions are briefly included in acknowledgements.

11.1.1　Acknowledgements writing

1. Object of acknowledgements

The object of acknowledgements mainly includes two kinds. One is the institutions that funded the study. The fund number should be indicated when referring to the source of funds. The second category is people who participated in part of the study without authorship.

2. Requirements and format of acknowledgements

Different SCI journals have their own specific requirements for writing acknowledgements. Some journals，like *N Engl J Med*，*Nature* and *PNAS* (*Proceedings of the National Academy of Sciences*)，require authors to list acknowledgements and all or part of funding sources supporting the research for published papers. The following are some examples of several journals.

[**Sample 1—*N Engl J Med***] (**Geleris et al.，2020**)

Supported in part by grants (RO1-LM006910，RO1-HL077612，RO1-HL093081，and RO1-HL121270) from the National Institutes of Health.

Disclosure forms provided by the authors are available with the full text of this article at NEJM. org.

We acknowledge the dedication，commitment，and sacrifice of the staff，providers，and personnel in our institution through the Covid-19 crisis and the suffering and loss of our patients as well as in their families and our community.

[**Sample 2—*Nature***] (**Hyland et al. , 2020**)

Acknowledgements

Funding for this work was provided by the Swiss National Science Foundation (Grant No. 176005 to G. R. and T. M. M. and SNSF Starting Grant No. 155913 to K. B.). G. R., S. L. H. and K. B. received core funding from ETH Zürich. We gratefully acknowledge the helpful discussions with H. Strathmann and V. Gal. We thank V. Andreas, X. Bonilla, D. Sidebotham, N. Toussaint and I. Jarchum for proofreading the manuscript.

[**Sample 3—*PNAS***] (**Abraham, 2017**)

ACKNOWLEDGEMENTS. We thank Dr. Can Bruce for microbiota sequence analysis, Michael Schadt for excellent technical assistance with histology, Huihui Dong for technical assistance with assorted in vitro experiments, and Morven Graham (Yale School of Medicine, Center for Cellular and Molecular Imaging) for help with the microscopic imaging. We thank William Gray and Bradley Parry for critical input on the analysis strategy for the fluorescence microscopy. The S. aureus WTA mutants were provided by Dr. Andreas Peschel (University of Tubingen, Tubingen, Germany). This work was supported, in part, by a gift from the John Monsky and Jennifer Weis Monsky Lyme Disease Research Fund. The F. C. laboratory received funding support from Laboratory for Molecular Infection Medicine Sweden, Knut and Alice Wallenberg Foundation, Kempe and the Swedish Research Council (VR). A. K. Y. was supported by a Umeå Center for Microbial Research/VR postdoctoral position. This work was supported by National Institutes of Health Grant 41440. E. F. and C. J.-W. are investigators of the Howard Hughes Medical Institute.

It is requested by *Science* journals that acknowledgements should include funding information, authors' contributions, a description of conflicts of interest, and data and materials availability. In the Instructions for Preparing an Initial Manuscript, *Science* details its writing requirements for the acknowledgements as follows:

> **Acknowledgements** should be gathered into a paragraph after the final numbered reference. This section should start by acknowledging non-author contributions, and then should provide information under the following headings. **Funding:** include complete funding information; **Authors contributions:** a complete list of contributions to the paper (we encourage you to follow the CRediT model). **Competing interests:** competing interests of any of the authors must be listed (all authors must also fill out the Conflict of Interest Form). Where authors have no competing interests, this should also be declared. **Data and materials availability:** any restrictions on materials such as MTAs. Accession numbers to any data relating to the paper and deposited in a public database. If all data is in

the paper and supplementary materials include the sentence "all data is available in the manuscript or the supplementary materials." (All data, code, and materials used in the analysis must be available to any researcher for purposes of reproducing or extending the analysis.)

[**Sample 4—*Science***] (**Yu**, **2020**)

ACKNOWLEDGEMENTS

We thank D. Lauffenburger, T. Orekov, A. Thomas, M. Porto, N. Thornburg, P. Abbink, E. Borducchi, M. Silva, A. Richardson, C. Caron, and J. Cwiak for generous advice, assistance, and reagents. **Funding**: We acknowledge support from the Ragon Institute of MGH, MIT, and Harvard, Mark and Lisa Schwartz Foundation, Beth Israel Deaconess Medical Center, Massachusetts Consortium on Pathogen Readiness (MassCPR), Janssen Vaccines & Prevention BV, and the National Institutes of Health (OD024917, AI129797, AI124377, AI128751, AI126603 to D. H. B.; AI007151 to D. R. M.; AI146779 to A. G. S.; AI121394, AI139538 to D. R. W.; 272201700036I - 0 - 759301900131 - 1, AI100625, AI110700, AI132178, AI149644, AI108197 to R. S. B.). We also acknowledge a Burroughs Wellcome Fund Postdoctoral Enrichment Program Award to D. R. M. **Author contributions**: D. H. B. designed the study. J. Y., L. H. T., L. P., N. B. M., K. M., S. H. M., J. P. N., J. L., Z. L., A. C., E. A. B., G. D., M. S. G., X. H., C. J. D., M. K., N. K., Z. L., L. F. M., F. N., R. N., J. V., and H. W. performed the immunologic and virologic assays. D. R. M. and R. S. B. performed the live virus neutralization assays. C. L., C. A., S. F., J. S. B., M. D. S., and G. A. performed the systems serology. Y. C., A. Z., F. J. N. L., M. T., S. H., and D. R. W. provided the convalescent human specimens. L. P., A. V. R., K. B., R. B., A. C., B. F., A. D., E. T., J. D. V., H. A., and M. G. L. led the clinical care of the animals. R. Z. and F. W. participated in study design and interpretation of data. Y. C., B. C., and A. G. S. provided purified proteins. D. H. B., J. L., Z. L., and B. C. designed the immunogens. D. H. B. wrote the paper with all co-authors. **Competing interests**: The authors declare no competing financial interests. D. H. B. is a co-inventor on related vaccine patents. R. Z. and F. W. are employees of Janssen Vaccines & Prevention BV. **Data and materials availability**: All data are available in the manuscript or the supplementary materials. Correspondence and requests for materials should be addressed to D. H. B. (dbarouch@bidmc.harvard.edu).

11.1.2 Contributions writing

Many SCI journals have strict regulations on the qualifications of authors. It is required to indicate the specific contribution of each author to this study when submitting the paper. In 2012, CRediT (Contributor Roles Taxonomy) was introduced to journals and authors, with the intention of sharing an accurate and detailed description of the authors' diverse contributions to the published work, reducing authorship disputes and facilitating collaboration. CRediT statements should be provided during the submission process and will appear above the acknowledgements section of the published paper. In some journals, actually, the acknowledgements are often followed by the contributions.

CRediT suggests a category of the listed role(s) or contributions of all authors as: conceptualization, methodology, software designing, validation, formal analysis, investigation, resources, data curation, writing—original draft, writing—review & editing, visualization, supervision, project administration, funding acquisition.

[**Sample 5**—*Nature*] (**Hyland et al. , 2020**)

Author contributions

S. L. H. , M. Hüser, X. L. , M. F. , G. R. , T. M. M. , K. B. , T. G. designed the experiments; M. F. , T. M. M. selected and provided the clinical data and context; X. L. , M. F. , S. L. H, M. Hüser with contributions from T. M. M. , M. Z. and G. R. preprocessed and cleaned the data; S. L. H. , M. F. , T. M. M. with contributions from G. R. , X. L. , M. Hüser defined and developed the labeling of deterioration events; M. Hüser, M. F. , with contributions from X. L. , S. L. H. , T. M. M. , G. R. devised and implemented the adaptive imputation strategy; M. Hüser, M. F. , X. L. , S. L. H. developed and extracted non-shapelet features, T. G. and C. B. developed code for shapelet analysis; M. Hüser, X. L. , S. L. H. developed the pipeline for supervised learning; X. L. implemented the LSTM model; T. G. implemented the decision tree baseline. C. E. , C. B. , M. F. , M. Horn, M. M. , B. R. , D. B. contributed to various analyses of the data; T. M. M. , G. R. , S. L. H. , M. F. , K. B. conceived and directed the project; S. L. H. , M. F. , M. Hüser, X. L. , T. G. , T. M. M. , G. R. , K. B. wrote the manuscript with the assistance and feedback of all the other co-authors. S. L. H. and T. G. with input from all authors created Fig. 1.

11.2　References and citation style

11.2.1　Reasons for referencing

Referencing is a standardized format and style of acknowledging sources of information and ideas that you have used in your article. There are a number of reasons for referencing sources. For example, you should acknowledge the source to show where your idea originated. Another reason for referencing is to give your writing academic weight, i.e., to show that you have carried out research and found evidence for your viewpoint. You also need to show that you are aware of the opinions or views expressed by other writers in the field. Finally, it is important to allow the readers to find the original source if necessary. Omitting to reference your sources, thus failing to acknowledge other people's ideas, is considered to be plagiarism. This is unaccepted in an academic piece of work (McCormack & Slaght, 2015). Therefore, referencing is necessary to show your academic attitude, to present your knowledge and understanding of your research, to verify quotations, to avoid plagiarism, to indicate the significance of your research, and to enable readers to follow-up and read more fully the cited author's arguments.

11.2.2　Types of referencing

Citing a source is a two-step process. The first one is in-text citation. It refers to the author by surname and the date of publication at the end of a borrowed information within your essay. The second one is bibliography. It is a list of references on the last page of your essay, with detailed information for each source. (McCormack & Slaght, 2015)

11.2.3　Referencing steps

1. Note down the full bibliographic details such as authors/editors, article/journal title, edition, volume(issue) number, place of publication, publisher, year of publication, and database name or web address, etc.

2. Insert the in-text citations in the appropriate place within the text of your article by editing the noted bibliographic details to a standard in-text citation.

3. Provide a reference list after the article text by editing the noted bibliographic details to a standard format.

11.2.4　Common in-text citation/note of medical academic article

The in-text citation of medical academic paper/article is in American Medical

Association (AMA) citation style. In in-text citation AMA style, reference items must be numbered consecutively in the order they are cited in the text. When citing the same source more than once, give the number of the original reference. Multiple sources can be listed at a single reference point. The multiple citation numbers are separated by commas and consecutive numbers are joined with a hyphen, using superscript numbers, e. g.[7-9,15,16], or standard numbers in brackets, e. g. (7 - 9,15, 16). In addition, strictly speaking, superscript numbers are placed outside periods and commas, and inside colons and semicolons.

In this way, AMA in-text citations can keep the text smooth and brief so that the readers can read more easily. The readers can also check the references according to the matched in-text citation if they are interested and want to get more information about this source.

Here is an example of an in-text citation and of its corresponding entry in the works-cited list. Notice the position and punctuation of the citation—at the end of the last sentence of the borrowed information, before the final period.

[Sample 6—Citation in superscript]

Case-control studies have reported positive associations between ever use of powder in the genital area and ovarian cancer, with an estimated odds ratio of 1. 24 in a pooled analysis[4] and 1. 31 in a meta-analysis.[5] However, these findings may be affected by recall bias,[6,7] and a recent surge in talc-related lawsuits and media coverage[8,9] has increased this possibility. Thus, it is crucial to evaluate the talc-ovarian cancer association using prospective data.

To date, three large cohort studies have assessed the association between use of powder in the genital area and ovarian cancer risk, with inconsistent results.[10-12] (O'Brien, 2020)

[Sample 7—Citation in parentheses]

Defining whether humans can naturally develop cross-immunity requires investigation (11). At present, studies using sera from individuals who have recovered from SARS or COVID-19 infections have shown limited cross-neutralization, suggesting that recovery from one infection does not protect against the other (12). (Weiddleder, 2020)

11.2.5 Bibliography in AMA citation style

Citation style depends on the subject matter. You may be required to use a particular citation style. Generally, three kinds of source style are used in academic researches for reference guidelines: AMA (American Medical Association) for medicine, health, and biological sciences, APA (American Psychological Association) for psychology, education, and other social sciences, MLA (Modern Language Association of American) for humanities including literature, arts, and history, etc. Here, we only discuss AMA.

11.2.5.1　A brief introduction to AMA format

The AMA format is a product of the format and style that standardized medical journal reference reports in the United States in the second half of the 20th century. The full name of the AMA is American Medical Association Manual of Style. Medical or health-related articles cited in reference are usually in AMA format. Some basic rules for most common citation styles are readily available online. For special requirements of reference formats and style of specific journals, search the web pages of relevant journals. Although each SCI journal and its series of journals have a fixed reference format, even within the same journal, different types of reference formats can vary in some places. In general, medical references adopt or are based on AMA format. The following section discusses the general format of the AMA.

11.2.5.2　General rules for referencing

According to the 10th edition of *AMA Citation Style*, there are some general rules to follow when referencing.

- Reference items must be listed numerically in the order they are cited in the text;
- Authors could be included up to 6;
- For more than six authors, provide the first three authors' names and then add "et al." (sometimes the first author followed by "et al." actually);
- If there is no author, start with the title;
- Titles of periodical (journals, magazines, and newspapers) should be abbreviated according to common and proper usage;
- Use the right punctuation;
- The order of details in the reference is correct.

11.2.5.3　Referencing journal or magazine article in AMA

In AMA citation style, the reference list is arranged numerically in the order in which references are cited in the text.

1. Journal or magazine article-in print

In the bibliography of a journal article, the details required include: authors, title of the article, title of the journal, volume and issue number of the journal, year of publication, and page numbers.

Authors should be listed with their last names first, followed by initials of their first names, and the authors are separated by commas and the last author is followed by a full stop. Usually, for papers with more than three authors, include only the first three authors' names or the first author's name followed by "et al.". Titles of articles cited in reference lists should be in upright with the first word of the title capitalized，and the title must be written exactly as it appears in the work cited，ending with a full stop. Journal titles are usually italic and abbreviated according to common usage （followed by a full stop），then the publication year （followed by a semicolon），volume numbers followed by journal issue in bracket （followed by a colon），finally the full inclusive pages of the article ending with a full stop.

To make it easier，the above details are generalized as following arrangement. Pleases pay attention to some details such as capitalization，italic，parenthesis，punctuation and the place of "et al." Referencing journal or magazine article in print in AMA citation can be simplified as the following template：

- **Journal article with 1 - 6 authors**：first author's last Name（第一作者姓） first Name initial（第一作者名的首字母），second author's last Name first Name initial. Article title（文章标题）. *Journal Title*（杂志名）. year of publication（出版年）；volume（卷号）（issue）（期号）：page numbers （参考页码）.

- **Journal article with more than 6 authors**：first author's last Name（第一作者姓） first Name initial（第一作者名的首字母），second author's last Name first Name initial，third author's last Name first Name initial，et al. Article title（文章标题）. *Journal Title* （杂志名）. year of publication（出版年）；volume（卷号）（issue）（期号）：page numbers（参考页码）.

［**Sample 8—With 1 author**］
Berkley S. Make vaccine coverage a key UN health indicator. *Nature*. 2015；526 （7572）：165 - 168.

［**Sample 9—With 2 - 6 authors**］
Myburgh JA，Mythen MG. Resuscitation fluids. *N Engl J Med*. 2013；369（13）：1243 - 1251.

［**Sample 10—With more than 6 authors**］
Hoffmann M，Kleine-Weber H，Schroeder S，et al. SARS-CoV-2 cell entry depends on ACE2 and TMPRSS2 and is blocked by a clinically proven protease inhibitor. *Cell*. 2020；181（2）：271 - 280.

2. Journal article-online

For online articles，authors，article title，journal name and the year of publication should be given as above，followed by DOI （digital object identifier）. If there is no DOI，provide the URL for the specific article.

［**Sample 11**］
Verheij J，van Lingen A，Beishuizen A，et al. Cardiac response is greater for colloid than saline fluid loading after cardiac or vascular surgery. *Intensive Care Med*. 2006；32（7）：1030 - 1038. doi：10. 1007/s00134 - 006 - 0195 - 5

11.2.5.4 Referencing books in print in AMA

In the case of a book, author lists should be given as above of cited articles. Book titles should be italic with the first word of the title capitalized, ending with a full stop, then place of publication (followed by a colon), publisher (followed by a semicolon), and year of publication (with a full stop).

For article or chapter in a book, the name of the article or the title of the chapter should be in upright with the first word of the title capitalized. Referencing books in AMA citation can be simplified as the following template:

- **Entire book with 1 – 6 author(s)**: first author's last Name(第一作者姓) first Name initial(第一作者名的首字母), second author's last Name(第二作者姓) first Name initial(第二作者名的首字母), the last author's last Name(最后作者姓) first Name(最后作者名的首字母). *Book Title*(书名). Place of publication (出版地): Publisher(出版社); year of publication(出版年).

- **Entire book with more than 3 or 6 authors** (it depends): the first author's last Name(第一作者姓) first Name initial(第一作者名的首字母), the second author's last Name(第二作者姓) first Name initial(第二作者名的首字母), the third author's last Name(第三作者姓) first Name initial(第三作者名的首字母), et al. *Book Title*(书名). Place of publication(出版地): Publisher(出版社); year of publication (出版年).

- **An Article or chapter in a book**: the author's last Name(作者姓) first Name initial (作者名的首字母). Article/Chapter title. (文章/标题). In: book author's last Name(书作者姓) first Name initial(书作者名的首字母), ed/s. *Book Title*(书名). Place of publication(出版地): Publisher(出版社); year of publication(出版年): page numbers(参考页码).

[Sample 12—Entire book with 1 author]

Zeiger M. *Essentials of Writing Biomedical Research Papers* 2nd ed. New York: McGraw Hill Co.; 2006.

[Sample 13—Entire book with 2 – 6 authors]

Modlin J, Jenkins P. *Decision Analysis in Planning for a Polio Outbreak in the United States*. San Francisco, CA: Pediatric Academic Societies; 2004.

[Sample 14—Entire book with more than 6 authors]

Rodgers P, Smith K, Williams D, Jones A, Brown W, Green B, et al. *The Way Forward for Australian Libraries*. Perth: Wombat Press; 2002.

[Sample 15—Entire book with more than 3 authors]

Aronoff GR, Berns JS, Brier ME, et al. *Drug Prescribing in Renal Failure* 4th ed. Philadelphia, PA: American College of Physicians; 1999.

[Sample 16—A chapter in a book]

Solensky R. Drug allergy：desensitization and treatment of reactions to antibiotics and aspirin. In：Lockey P，ed. *Allergens and Allergen Immunotherapy* 3rd ed. New York，NY：Marcel Dekker；2004：585 – 606.

[Sample 17—Entire book without any author]

Oxford dictionary for scientific writers and editors. Oxford：Clarendon；1991.

11.2.5.5 Website references in AMA

The first part is the title of notice，followed by the website to show where it appeared. The dates refer to when it is published，updated，or reviewed.

E-documents（电子文献著录格式）

the author's last Name（作者姓）first Name initial（作者名的首字母）. Title（题名）[EB/OL]（电子文献/载体类型标识）. the source of E-documents（电子文献的出处），update date/reference date（发表或更新日期/引用日期）.

[Sample 18]

2014 – 2016 Ebola outbreak in West Africa[EB/OL]. Centers for Disease Control and Prevention Website. http：//www. cdc. gov/vhf/ebola/outbreaks/2014-west-africa/index. html，March 8，2019 / October 20，2020.

Chapter Review

This unit has mainly discussed how to write contributions and acknowledgements，and how to make in-text citation and references for English medical academic articles. The learners are expected：

1. to write appropriate and standard acknowledgements and contributions for your paper；

2. to understand the reasons for referencing；

3. to know the types and functions of referencing；

4. to practice how to prepare references under referencing steps；

5. to be able to make in-text citations in the text of medical academic papers；

6. to be able to make references in AMA format and style.

Assignments

Task 1 *Read the reference entry and answer the following questions.*

O'Brien KM，Tworoger SS，Harris HR，et al. Association of powder in the genital area with risk of ovarian cancer. *JAMA*. 2020；323（1）：49 – 59. doi：10. 1001/jama. 2019. 20079

a. Who are the authors of the article?

b. Are the three authors arranged by the alphabetical order of the initial letters in surnames?

c. When was the article published?

d. What is the title of the article?

e. Where was the article published?

f. Which page is referenced?

g. What's the website of this essay?

Task 2 *Use the AMA citation style to write references for papers 1 – 7 in Appendix Ⅱ. You can find relevant information from the article page.*

Task 3 *Study the acknowledgements and contributions of the papers in Appendix Ⅱ. Then discuss the factors that should be included in acknowledgements and contributions with your partners, and try to write acknowledgements and contributions for your paper or for your supposed paper in the future.*

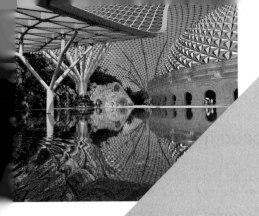

Chapter Twelve

Common Errors in English Academic Paper Writing

Lead-in Questions

What do you know about the role of language in academic papers?

Learning Objectives

After learning this unit, you will be able to:

1. understand the importance of language in English academic paper writing,

2. identify the common language errors in journal articles,

3. and make practices in adapting the linguistic norms in English academic article.

✓参考答案
✓课件申请
✓学术资源

12.1 Language of English academic papers

English academic papers submitted for publication are now facing intense competition for limited space of a journal, and therefore most papers are likely to be rejected. The rejection of submitted manuscripts may be caused by non-content elements, such as poor formatting, writing style, language, and outdated references. This chapter draws on an article entitled "Primary Caregivers and Chinese Elders' Demand on Community Services" (Zhang, 2020) as an example to illustrate the importance of language in journal article writing and some common types of errors occurring in papers.

The first version of this article was rejected by the journal *Social Service Research*. Martin Hyde, the Deputy Editor of the journal, commented: "To be frank, the author has not given adequate context of community-based eldercare services in China. The translation of 'community-based in-home services' or other is directly from Mandarin, which can be confusing to readers who are not familiar with long-term care in China." A lack of clarity in expressions seems a major reason for its rejection.

Substantially revised by a colleague of the author, a language teacher, the new version of this article was accepted and finally published by the journal in 2020. This case indicates that language is vital to English academic paper writing. By analyzing some revisions of the paper, this chapter discusses the language errors commonly occurring in English academic paper writing.

12.2 Common language errors in English academic paper writing

12.2.1 Comma errors

English comma (,) can be used in two ways: 1) to connect words or phrases such as "mistake, misrepresentation, duress, and failure of consideration"; "spouses, daughters-in-law and daughters"; 2) to connect sentences/clauses with conjunctions (e.g., but, and, for, or, if, when, because, since). Yet when only a comma is used to connect two independent clauses, a comma splice, a grammatical mistake, will occur. This type of error can be corrected by using either a semicolon or a period instead. Strunk and White (2007) states, "If two or more clauses, grammatically complete and not joined by a conjunction, are to form a single compound sentences, the proper mark of punctuation is a semicolon or period. " (see Samples 1 – 2)

[Sample 1]

This amendment is the most important source of limitations on the states' power over individuals; most of the protections of the Bill of Rights are application to the states.

[Sample 2]

This amendment is the most important source of limitations on the states' power over individuals. Most of the protections of the Bill of Rights are application to the states.

[Analysis]

If the second clause is preceded by an adverb, such as "accordingly", "besides", "then", "therefore", or "thus", a conjunction should be used. Do not combine independent clauses merely with a comma. Otherwise, an error occurs as in Sample 3.

[Sample 3]

Second, elders cared for by daughters-in-law tend to seek more community care, therefore they should be the priority for community services in China.

[Analysis] In Sample 3, a grammatical error occurs by a misused comma in that a comma itself cannot connect two independent sentences. The word "therefore" is an adverb rather than a conjunction. The conjunction "and" can be added to correct the error, as in Revision.

[Revision] Second, elders cared for by daughters-in-law tend to seek more community care, and therefore, they should be the priority for community services in China.

[Analysis] In Sample 3, the grammatical error is caused by misplaced punctuations, and adverbs are mistakenly used as conjunctions, as in the following examples: "Hiring a cleaner enchants their daily life, then it could be an optimal choice / Having net friends requires more time to be spent in front of computer, thus adolescents apply less time to former friends and participate in less outdoor activities".

12.2.2 Grammatical errors

1. Dangling modifiers

Dangling modifiers are a common type of grammatical errors made by learners or even scholars. A dangling modifier, also known as "dangling participles", "hanging modifier", or "floating modifiers", is an error caused by failing to use the word that the modifier is meant to be modifying. Though dangling modifiers sometimes occur because writers assume what they're talking about is so obvious from the context that they forget to mention it, using a dangling modifier will tell your readers that you have an unfirm grasp of grammar and that you're not a clear thinker. Dangling modifiers cause the unclear meaning of a sentence (see Sample 4).

[**Sample 4**]

Accordingly, a simple generalization of findings to all societies is problematic when interpreting the elderly's need of formal services.

[**Analysis**] The modifier "when interpreting the elderly's need of formal services" is correctly used only when the agent has the ability to interpret. Yet the fact that the subject of the sentence, i. e. "a simple generalization of findings", is unable to interpret, which leads to the dangling modifier. To correct this error, the when-clause can be replaced by a prepositional phrase like "as to the interpretation of the elderly's need of formal services", as in Revision.

[**Revision**] Accordingly, a simple generalization of findings to all societies is problematic as to the interpretation of the elderly's need of formal services.

2. Tense errors

Keep a consistent use of tense(s) whenever necessary within the same sentence or paragraph. Shifting from one tense to another without a good reason often causes confusion and distraction. "In summarizing, use the present tense. Shifting from one tense to another gives the appearance of uncertainty and irresolution" (Strunk & White, 2007). Yet this convention is sometimes violated in novice writers' writing, as in Sample 5.

[**Sample 5**]

However, past studies showed that only a small proportion of elders and caregivers have taken advantage of these community services.

[**Analysis**] A tense shift, from past tense to present perfect, occurs in the above complex sentence. It is better to keep a consistent use of tense(s) except that a tense shift can be justified, as in Revision.

[**Revision**] However, past studies have showed that only a small proportion of elders and caregivers have taken advantage of these community services.

12.2.3 Redundancy

Vigorous writing of an academic paper should be concise from title, abstract to main text. For example, it is indicated in the instructions for preparing an initial manuscript by *Science* that titles should be no more than 96 characters (including spaces), and that the abstract should be 125 words or less. This means that all the information included in the paper should be brief and concise. A redundant sentence contains unnecessary words; a redundant paragraph includes unnecessary sentences. Strunk and White (2007) present some examples as follows:

the question as to whether→whether (the question whether)

there is no doubt but that→no doubt (doubtless)

he is a man who→he

this is a subject that→this subject

[Sample 6]

It means that the covariates drawn from the theoretical model do have significant influence but the direction of the influence on Chinese elders' demand on community services is altered.

[Analysis] In Sample 6, unnecessary words "It means that" make the wording redundant. In Revision, "It means that" is replaced by a more concise expression, "Specifically".

[Revision] Specifically, the covariates drawn from the theoretical model do have significant influence but the direction of the influence on Chinese elders' demand on community services is altered.

[Sample 7]

China, the country with the largest population in the world, is also the country that has the most elderly people in the globe.

[Analysis]

In Sample 7, the superfluous expressions such as "the country", "also the country", "the world", and "the globe" can be omitted, as in Revision.

[Revision]

China, heavily populated in the world, is also dense with elderly people.

12.3   Common errors in coherence and cohesion

A unified paragraph maintains coherence and unity, with a central idea controlling the paragraph. The central idea can be presented in the topic sentence at the beginning of the paragraph, followed by supporting sentences which develop cases and evidences related to the central idea. This approach of paragraph development is often applied to journal article writing. This section presents some errors related to the violation of this convention.

12.3.1   Common errors in coherence

Incoherence usually occurs in a paragraph with an incomplete topic sentence (Sample 8) or without a topic sentence (Samples 9 – 10).

[**Sample 8**]

The contributions of the research are: First, traditional Anderson and Newman's model can be applied toelucidate Chinese elderly's "demand" on community services. Second, elders cared for by daughters-in-law tend to seek more community care, therefore they should be the priority for community services in China.

[**Analysis**] Without a topic sentence, the paragraph of Sample 8 is not well organized. The first sentence in the paragraph can be changed to a topic sentence, as shown in Revision.

[**Revision**] The current research has two contributions to future study in related areas. First, traditional Anderson and Newman's model can be applied to elucidate Chinese elderly's "demand" on community services. Second, elders cared for by daughters-in-law tend to seek more community care, and therefore, they should be the priority for community services in China.

[**Sample 9**]

Undoubtedly, such a huge elderly population will have a strong demand on daily care and services. With a deep root of Confucianism, traditional care of elder people in China has been provided at home by spouses, adult children, children-in-laws (particularly daughters-in-law) and extended family members (Wu, 2005; Zhan, 2003). Since 1979 when China launched the family planning policy (One Child policy), traditional extended family caregiving networks has been greatly challenged due to declining fertility and a dramatic increase of empty nest households. The economic reforms after the 1980s also pushed a tremendous amount of rural people to leave their hometown and rush to cities for better paid jobs. All these changes have made it difficult for older people to remain receiving sufficient care from their families (Poston, 2000).

[**Analysis**] Due to a lack of unity, Sample 9 is difficult to understand. To enhance the paragraph coherence, a topic sentence ("The traditional care of elder people in China are facing two major policy challenges") can be added after the background of the discussed issue is introduced, as in Revision.

[**Revision**] With a deep root of Confucianism, traditional care of elder people in China has been provided at home by spouses, adult children, children-in-laws (particularly daughters-in-law) and extended family members (Wu et al., 2005; Zhan & Montgomery, 2003). The traditional care of elder people in China are facing two major policy challenges. This first case is a family policy since 1979 when China launched the family planning policy (One Child policy). Traditional extended family caregiving networks have been greatly challenged due to declining fertility and a dramatic increase of empty nest households. The second one is that the economic reforms after the 1980s also pushed a tremendous amount of rural people to leave their hometown and rush to cities for better paid jobs. All these changes have made it difficult for older people to remain receiving sufficient care from their families (Poston & Duan, 2000). Undoubtedly, such a huge elderly population will have a strong demand on daily care and services.

[**Sample 10**]

During the past few decades, although researchers have modified Anderson and Newman's framework by including predisposing, enabling needs and characteristics of care recipients and primary caregivers (Bass & Noelker, 1987), most studies focused exclusively on studying the elderly's characteristics and needs, and they neglected the situation of caregivers.

[**Analysis**] Poorly organized, Sample 10 is hard to understand. A topic sentence is added in Revision to enhance coherence. Moreover, the tense shifting problem in Sample 10 ("have modified", "neglected") is solved in Revision ("have modified", "have neglected").

[**Revision**] The past few decades have witnessed two achievements in this field. In the first case researchers have modified Anderson and Newman's framework by including predisposing, enabling needs and characteristics of care recipients and primary caregivers (Bass & Noelker, 1987). Moreover, they focused their studies exclusively on studying the elderly's characteristics and needs. However, they have neglected the situation of caregivers.

12.3.2 Common errors in cohesion

Cohesion is achieved by syntactical features such as deictic, anaphoric and cataphoric elements or logical tense structures. There are two main types of cohesion: grammatical cohesion, and lexical cohesion. Cohesive errors are often caused by topic shifts, as in Samples 11 – 12.

[**Sample 11**]

Please note that since almost all elders who were cared for by unmarried sons and daughters reported needing home care services, when the primary caregiver variable is used to predict the respondent's need of home care services, the regression coefficient is automatically omitted by the statistical software. Thus, the table shows " – " to represent the omitted regression coefficients.

[**Analysis**] In Sample 11, the topic of the passage shifts from the second person pronoun "you" (implied in the sentence) to the third person perspective "the table". A possible revision is to replace "Please note that" with "These following facts need to be noticed".

[**Sample 12**]

To promote utilization of home-based community services, it is essential to investigate who seeks assistance from the community and what factors have pushed the elderly to do so. Using a national sample of non-institutionalized elders from Chinese Longitudinal Health and Longevity Surveys (CLHLS), this research focuses on investigating how primary caregiver relationships with the elderly predict Chinese elderly's demand on community services. The next section of the paper will review the theoretical framework along with the existing literature.

[**Analysis**] In Sample 12, "To promote utilization …" indicates an action of purpose and its implied logic subject is person pronouns ("someone to promote"); however, both of the second and the last sentences use inanimate pronouns as their implied logic subjects ("this research", "The next section of the paper"), and the last sentence expresses other action of purpose. The topic shifts in the three sentences make the readers confused to understand the text clearly.

[**Revision**] The beginning infinitive phrase "To promote utilization of home-based community services" can be changed to a prepositional phrase "In the utilizing promotion of home-based community services".

12.4 Plagiarism in writing English academic papers

Plagiarism originates from the Latin word *plagiarius*, meaning "kidnapper". When one uses other people's words or ideas as one's own without properly acknowledging the original sources, he/she may commit plagiarism. Though plagiarism is a complex academic phenomenon, it is generally acceptable if authors appropriately re-use other scholars' ideas or expressions through making paraphrases or summaries and give credit to these cited sources. To avoid plagiarism in academic paper writing, it is also necessary for student writers to learn how to cite academic references.

12.4.1 General types of plagiarism

Plagiarism is not a pure black-and-white issue. On some occasions, the repetition of certain textual phrases without documentation may not be considered as plagiarism, such as standardized expressions (e. g., "boilerplate"). Yet the following behaviors can be regarded as plagiarism:

- Copying large sections of others' materials and claiming them as your own.
- Translating from another language without acknowledging the source.
- Imitating a textual structure or an argument without attribution.
- Changing sources by replacing or altering vocabulary and syntax.
- Reproducing or modifying source text without crediting the author.

- Taking others' ideas as your own.
- Quoting references without attribution.
- Reporting some academic information and figures from other papers without attribution.
- Writing a lab report with a method section borrowed from a published paper.
- Blending some source materials into a report.
- Presenting the ideas, work or words of other people without any acknowledgement.
- Submitting work that you have presented for assessment on a previous occasion.
- Submitting materials from "essay banks".
- Copying another student's work.

12.4.2   Samples and analysis

Copying others' words without any changes can lead to plagiarism, especially at the sentential level and paragraph level (Sample 13).

[Sample 13]

According to Hinkel (2004: 1), extensive, thorough, and focused instruction in L2 academic vocabulary, grammar, and discourse is essential for developing L2 written proficiency.

[Analysis] As the sentence in Sample 13 is a direct copy of the source text, thus causing plagiarism. The sentence needs to be restated with the user's own words, as in Revision.

[Revision] L2 written proficiency is expected to be thoroughly trained in L2 class instruction via academic vocabulary, grammar and discourse (Hinkel, 2004).

The revision involves paraphrasing. A paraphrase helps reconstruct the original text by transforming its lexis and syntactic structures. An improper paraphrase is only done with partial changes like lexical changes " ... are essential to ... → ... are essentially vital/important/... " A proper paraphrase needs the reconstruction of the original source text in a fresh way as in Revision.

12.4.3   Methods to avoid plagiarism

1. Document paraphrased sources

The key method to avoid plagiarism is to acknowledge and document the sources you use. Different disciplines use different documentation styles, for instance, MLA style for literature papers, APA style or other "date-first" style for qualitative or quantitative research papers, and AMA for medicine, health, and biological sciences.

2. Summarizing or paraphrasing

On the premise of documenting paraphrased sources, authors should use their own words to summarize or paraphrase the source text to avoid plagiarism. It is also helpful to draft your academic papers with reference to your reading notes instead of the source text. When taking notes of the source text, make sure to:

- Understand the source text as fully as possible;
- Take notes based on your own understanding or summary.

Chapter Review

This chapter first discusses the common types of errors occurring in writing academic papers in English, namely comma errors, grammatical errors, redundancy, and errors in coherence and cohesion. In this chapter we have also discussed plagiarism and how to avoid it.

Assignments

Task 1   *List various forms of academic paper plagiarism you have noticed in this chapter.*

Task 2   *Give three strategies to avoid plagiarism in academic writing.*

a. _____ .
b. _____ .
c. _____ .

Task 3   *The following 15 sentences are mostly from Chinese scholars. Point out the errors of any kinds and then revise them.*

1. China, the country with the largest population in the world, is also the country that has the most elderly people in the globe.

2. Traditional extended family caregiving networks has been greatly challenged due to declining fertility and a dramatic increase of empty nest households.

3. However, past studies showed that only a small proportion of elders and caregivers have taken advantage of these community services.

4. To promote utilization of home-based community services, it is essential to investigate who seeks assistance from the community and what factors have pushed the elderly to do so.

5. The predisposing factors are conceptualized as factors existing prior to one's illness, which may affect the need for services but not necessarily be the cause of utilization.

6. During the past few decades, although researchers have modified Anderson and Newman's framework by including predisposing, enabling and need characteristics of care recipients and primary caregivers, most studies focused exclusively on studying the elderly's characteristics and needs, and they neglected the situation of caregivers.

7. Thus, the general findings of the existing literature were in Western countries, such as the U.S., elders cared for by their spouses alone tended to be more isolated and were less likely to rely on community services.

8. To measure need of community services, the research uses the survey question that asked the respondent: "What kind of social services do you expect to be provided by your community?"

9. Among the eight types of services, the elders reported home care services (77.7% of urban vs. 87.1% of rural), psychological consulting services (63.3% of urban vs. 65.1% of rural) and health care education services (73.1% of urban vs. 71.9% of rural) as their most desirable services.

10. Following a similar rationale, Table 3 – 1 is a full regression table that presents complete regression results for rural respondents.

11. This is because they differ greatly in role obligations to their care recipients and the context in which care is provided.

12. To impress the interviews, punctuality is essential.

13. After owning this special experience, it's easier and more comfortable for those young people to get along with colleagues after graduate.

14. Using a national sample of non-institutionalized elders from Chinese Longitudinal Health and Longevity Surveys (CLHLS), this research focuses on investigating how primary caregiver relationships with the elderly predict Chinese elderly's demand on community services.

15. Because people have changed and so have the instruments to achieve environment protection.

References

1. 黄一瑜,闵楠,殷红梅.医学院校硕士研究生英语读与写.第二版.北京:中国人民大学出版社,2008.

2. 詹姆斯·博尔顿,卢凤香,郭晶.医学 SCI 论文撰写与发表.北京:中国协和医科大学出版社,2016.

3. 吴江梅,黄佩娟.英语科技论文写作.北京:中国人民大学出版社,2015.

4. Alegre-Díaz J, Herrington W, Lopez-Cervantes M. et al. Diabetes and cause-specific mortality in Mexico city. *N Engl J Med*. 2016; 375(20): 1961-1971.

5. Abraham NM, Jutras BL, Yadav AK, et al. Pathogen-mediated manipulation of arthropod microbiota to promote infection. *Proc Natl Acad Soc*. 2017; 114 (5): E781-E790.

6. Ashraf RM. *Effective Technical Communication*. Tata: McGraw-Hill; 2005.

7. Bass DM, Noelker LS. The influence of family caregivers on elders use of in-home services: an expanded conceptual framework. *J Health Soc Behav*. 1987; 28: 184.

8. Brouter N, Krauer F, Riesen M, et al. Zika virus as a cause of neurologic disorders. *N Engl J Med*. 2016; 374 (16): 1506-1509.

9. Channell J. *Vague Language*. Oxford: Oxford University Press; 1994.

10. Crews F. *The Random House Handbook* 2nd ed. New York: Random House; 1977.

11. Danes F. Functional sentence perspective and the organization of the text. In: Danes F. ed. *Papers in Functional Sentence Perspective*. Prague: Academia; 1974.

12. Day RA. *How to Write and Publish a Scientific Paper* 5th ed. Arizona Phoenix: ORYX Press; 1998.

13. Day RA, Gastel B. *How to Write and Publish a Scientific Paper*. London: Greenwood Press; 2006.

14. Delabouglise A, Choisy M, Phan TD, et al. Economic factors influencing zoonotic disease dynamics: demand for poultry meat and seasonal transmission of avian influenza in Vietnam. *Sci Rep*. 2017; 7: 1-14.

15. Ding ZH, Wang LL. Study on the equalization of home-based care services for the elderly in China. *Population J* (in Chinese). 2011; 5: 83-88.

16. Dwyer-Lindgren L, Cork MA, Sligar A, et al. Mapping HIV prevalence in sub-Saharan Africa between 2000 and 2017. *Nature*. 2019; 570: 189-195.

17. Evranos B, Aytemir K, Oto A, et al. Predictors of atrial fibrillation recurrence after atrial fibrillation ablation with cryoballoon. *Cardiol J*. 2013; 20(3): 294-303.

18. Guan W, Ni Z, Hu Y, et al. Clinical characteristics of coronoavirus disease 2019 in China. *N Engl J Med*. 2020; 18(3): 1708-1720.

19. Glendinning EH, Howard R. *Professional English in Use: Medicine*. Cambridge: Cambridge University Pres; 2009.

20. Gary B, Robert WB. *The Elements of Technical Writing*. New York: Macmillan Publishers; 1993.

21. Gehrig JI, Venkatesh S, Chang HW, et al. Effects of microbiota-directed foods in gnotobiotic animals and undernourished children. *Science*. 2019; 365: eaau4732.

22. Gierszewska K, Jaworska I, Skrzypek M, et al. Quality of life in patients with coronary artery disease treated with coronary artery bypass grafting and hybrid coronary revascularization. *Cardiol J*. 2018; 25(5): 621-627.

23. Haegeli LM, Stutz L, Mohsen M, et al. Feasibility of zero or near zero fluoroscopy during catheter ablation procedures. *Cardiol J*. 2019; 26(3), 226-232.

24. Halliday MAK. *An Introduction to Functional Grammar*. Beijing: Foreign language Teaching and Research Press; 2000.

25. Halliday MAK, Hasan R. *Cohesion in English*. Beijing: Foreign language Teaching and Research Press; 2001.

26. Hinkel E. *Second Language Writers' Text*. Malwah, New Jersey, and London: Lawrence Erlbaum Associates Publishers; 2002.

27. Hinkel E. *Teaching Academic ESL Writing, Practical Technique in Vocabulary and Grammar*. Malwah, New Jersey, and London: Lawrence Erlbaum Associates Publishers; 2004.

28. Huang X, Yin H, Yan L, et al. Epidemiological characteristics of HFRS in mainland China from 2006-2010. *WPSAR*. 2012 ; 3(1): 1-7.

29. Hyland K. The impact of teacher written feedback on individual writers. *J Second Language Writing*. 1998; 7(3): 255-286.

30. Hyland K. *English for Academic Purposes, An Advanced Resource Book*. Taylor & Francis Group: Routledge; 2006.

31. Isanaka S, Guindo O, Langendorf C, et al. Efficacy of a low-cost, heat-stable oral rotavirus vaccine in Niger. *N Engl J Med*. 2017; 376: 1121-1130.

32. Jetz W, Wilcove DS, Dobson AP. Projected impacts of climate and land-use change on the global diversity of birds. *PLoS Biol*. 2017; 5(6): e157.

33. Johnson NF, Velásquez N, Restrepo NJ, et al. The online competition between pro-and anti-vaccination views. *Nature*. 2020; https: //doi. org/10. 1038/s41586-020-2281-1.

34. Jordan A. *Text, Role, and Context: Developing Academic Literacies*. Cambridge: Cambridge University Press; 1997.

35. Kutyifa V, Rice J, Jones R, et al. Impact of non-cardiovascular disease burden on thirty-day hospital readmission in heart failure patients. *Cardio J*. 2018; 25(6): 691-700.

36. Kaplan R. Cultural thought patterns in inter-cultural education. *J Res in Language Studies*. 1966; 16: 11-25.

37. Katz MJ. *From Research to Manuscript: A Guide to Scientific Writing*. The Netherlands: Springer; 2006.

38. Langan, J. *College Writing Skills With Reading* 6th ed. Beijing: Foreign Language Teaching and Research Press; 2010.

39. Lewis M. *The Lexical Approach: the state of ELT and way forward*. Hove: Language Teaching Pub-lication; 1993.

40. Ledgerwood JE, DeZure AD, Stanley DA, et al. Chimpanzee adenovirus vector ebola vaccine. *N Engl J Med*. 2017; 376: 928-938.

41. Lu C, Black MM, Richter LM. Risk of poor development in young children in low- income and middle-income countries: an estimation and analysis at the global, regional, and country level. *Lancet Glob Health*. 2016; 4: e916-922.

42. Matthews BJ, Dudchenko O, Kingan SB, et al. Improved reference genome of Aedes aegypti informs arbovirus vector control. *Nature*. 2018; 563: 501 – 507.

43. Miyahara R, Takahashi K, Anh NTH, et al. Exposure to paternal tobacco smoking increased child hospitalization for lower respiratory infections but not for other diseases in Vietnam. *Sci Rep*. 2017; 7: 45481.

44. Nayagam S, Conteh L, Sicuri E, et al. Cost-effectiveness of community-based screening and treatment for chronic hepatitis B in the Gambia: an economic modelling analysis. *Lancet Glob Health*. 2016; 4: e568 – 578.

45. Ngonghala CN, De Leo GA, Pascual MM, et al. General ecological models for human subsistence, health and poverty. *Nature Ecol Evol*. 2017; 1: 1153 – 1159.

46. O'Brien KM, Tworoger SS, Harris HR, et al. Association of powder in the genital area with risk of ovarian cancer. *JAMA*. 2020; 323(1): 49 – 59.

47. Paules CI, Fauci AS. Yellow fever—once again on the radar screen in the Amercias. *New Engl J Med*. 2017; 376:1397 – 1399.

48. Poston D, Duan CR. The current and projected distribution of the elderly and eldercare in the People's Republic of China. *J Family Issues*. 2000; 21(6): 714 – 732.

49. Rosshart S, Herz J, Vassallo B, et al. Laboratory mice born to wild mice have natural microbiota and model human immune responses. *Science*. 2019; 365(6452): 444.

50. Rozakis LE. *Complete Idiot's Guide to Grammar and Style*. London: Penguin; 2003.

51. Sebranek P, Kemper D, Verne M. Writers. In: *A Student Handbook for Writing and Learning*. Wilmington: Houthton Mifflin Company; 2006.

52. Shi H, Han X, Jiang N, et al. Radiological findings from 81 patients with COVID-19 pneumonia in Wuhan, China: a descriptive study. *Lancet Infect Dis*. 2020; 20: 425 – 534.

53. Street SE, Navarrete AF, Reader SM, et al. Coevolution of cultural intelligence, extended life history, sociality, and brain size in primates. *Proc Natl Acad Sci*. 2017; 114(30): 7908 – 7914.

54. Strunk W Jr, White EB. *The Elements of Style* 4th ed. London: Penguin Books; 2007.

55. Swales JM, Feak CB. *Academic Writing for Graduate Students* 3rd ed. Michigan: University of Michigan Press; 2012.

56. The GBD 2015 Obesity Collaborators. Health effects of overweight and obesity in 195 countries over 25 years. *N Engl J Med*. 2017; 377(1): 13 - 27.

57. The GBD 2016 Lifetime Risk of Stroke Collaborators. Global, Regional, and Country-Specific Lifetime Risks of Stroke, 1990 and 2016. *N Engl J Med*. 2018; 379: 2429 – 2437.

58. Wang H, Wang Z, Dong Y, et al. Phase-adjusted estimation of the number of Coronavirus Disease 2019 cases in Wuhan, China. *Cell Discovery*. 2020; 6: 10 – 18.

59. Wang LL. A study on the demand, supply and utilization of home-based care services for the elderly based on the theory of "theory chain". *Population J* (in Chinese). 2013; 2: 49 – 53.

60. Webster's Seventh New Collegiate Dictionary. Springfield: G. & C. Merriam Company; 1969.

61. Weissleder R, Lee H, Ko J, et al. COVID-19 diagnostics in context. *Sci Transl Med*. 2020; 12 (3): eabc1931.

62. Wu B, Carter MW, Goins RT, et al. Emerging services for community-based long-term care in urban China: A systematic an63. alysis of Shanghai's community-based agencies. *J Ageing Soc Policy*. 2005; 17(4): 37 - 60.